YOGA FOR DEMENTIA

of related interest

Chair Yoga
Seated Exercises for Health and Wellbeing
Edeltraud Rohnfeld
ISBN 978 1 84819 078 8
eISBN 978 0 85701 056 8
DVD ISBN 978 1 84819 184 6

Qigong for Wellbeing in Dementia and Aging
Stephen Rath
Illustrated by LauRha Frankfort
ISBN 978 1 84819 253 9
eISBN 978 0 85701 199 2

'This book is a vital tool for people who are either living with dementia, caring for those living with dementia, or just travelling the aging pathway. The style (with its dip in, or read in full approach) makes it very accessible with good, clear and colourful illustrations. A marvellous opportunity to enhance lives.'

– Dr Lindesay M. C. Irvine, Senior Lecturer in Nursing, Queen Margaret University

'Tania has provided an easy-to-read and informative book. I am always striving for imaginative ways to keep residents moving and active. Tania's book provides practical and inspirational techniques authenticated by her own experiences. I recommend it for yoga novices young and old and anywhere in between.'

– Lisa Kieh, Plas Bryn Rhosyn Care Home Manager, Pobl Care

'Our yoga project was a great success, with very positive results for our clients living with dementia. I recommend that yoga is considered as a priority in the wellbeing and enjoyment of those within care, as it evidenced smiles, laughter and fun even for those who struggled to communicate. Thank you, Tania!'

– Maggie Candy, Care Home Manager

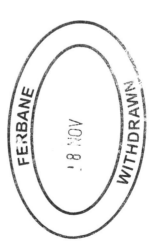

YOGA FOR

DEMENTIA

A Guide for People with Dementia, Their Families and Caregivers

Tania Plahay

Foreword by Martin Green

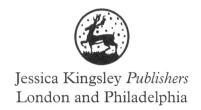

Jessica Kingsley *Publishers*
London and Philadelphia

First published in 2018
by Jessica Kingsley Publishers
73 Collier Street
London N1 9BE, UK
and
400 Market Street, Suite 400
Philadelphia, PA 19106, USA

www.jkp.com

Library of Congress Cataloging in Publication Data
A CIP catalog record for this book is available from the Library of Congress

British Library Cataloguing in Publication Data
A CIP catalogue record for this book is available from the British Library

ISBN 978 1 78592 159 9
eISBN 978 1 78450 433 5

Printed and bound in the UK

The videos can be accessed at www.jkp.com/voucher using the code PLAHAYYOGA.

This book has been inspired by my father, Narinder Singh Plahay, who passed away in 2001. Despite him not being physically here I regularly feel his guidance and consider him as being one of my greatest 'gurus' or teachers. Wherever his soul resides now, I hope that he would be proud of this book and my desire to help spread the power of yoga.

This book is also dedicated to my grandmother, Dorothea Collins, who passed away in the later stages of writing this book. She had been living with dementia for seven years. I wish I'd had the tools contained in this book while my grandmother was first living with dementia, as I feel they would have enabled me to understand what she was going through better and be more present with her.

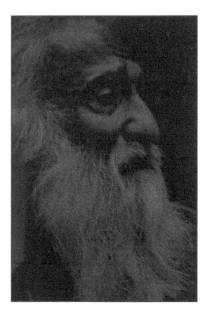
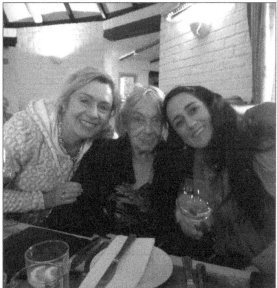

CONTENTS

FOREWORD

Professor Martin Green, Chief Executive, Care England, Department of Health and Independent Sector Dementia Champion

In the over 30 years that I have worked in social care, the populations of care homes have changed dramatically. In the past, care homes were often a lifestyle choice for older people who wanted companionship and some support with the activities of daily living. Today, care home residents have many more health conditions, and a large percentage of them are living with some form of dementia. The challenge for the care home sector of the 21st century is to ensure that people have a good quality of life, which will enable them to be as independent as possible. Of course, enabling people to live as long as they can safely and well within their own homes is also key, and this book provides many ways to allow people with early stage dementia to stay well for longer.

I am lucky enough to visit many care homes, and one of the things that I am really delighted to see is how creative and innovative this sector can be, and how it has embraced a range of new approaches that enable people to live well, maintain their independence, and continue to have good quality relationships with their families and friends.

The very best approaches look at the medical and social needs of people, and combine these together in a comprehensive approach, where people have the opportunity to connect with one another, whilst at the same time engaging in an activity that has really positive health benefits.

One of the best examples I have seen of all these things coming together, and making a real difference in the lives of care home residents, is yoga.

For many people who are not familiar with yoga, it is surrounded by myths and misconceptions, and this clouds their view about the benefits of yoga for those living with dementia. In this book, Tania Plahay brilliantly demystifies 'yoga', and clearly shows the different ways it can be used in care settings and homes, and the outstanding improvements in people's quality of life that can be achieved for residents.

The majority of people who live in care homes are taking a number of different drugs, and often these medical interventions, which are so important to controlling medical conditions, can also provide a range of side effects, which can leave people feeling lethargic and lacking in the desire or capacity to exercise.

There is also the added challenge for many people of coming to terms with moving into a care home because of a critical illness or frailty. This can often lead to anxiety and depression, and it is important that care services acknowledge this, and find creative ways to support people through their transition from living in their own home to a new life in a care setting.

This book works on so many levels, and gives a really clear route map on how to use yoga – as a group activity, as something that individuals can do for themselves, or as part of an individual and bespoke plan to keep people active and well. It also provides many activities that can be done together with family members or carers, which will benefit all those involved.

What is also great about this book is its applicability to so many people who might be at different stages of either physical or cognitive impairment. Yoga is a great way of releasing stress and anxiety, and can be used as a positive way of supporting people who might have a relatively new diagnosis of dementia and are coming to terms with what this will mean for their lives. It is also a great way of connecting with people who are living with dementia and who have significant cognitive impairments. Yoga really can help everyone in the care home setting and those living in their own homes, and Tania explains various ways that care providers and family carers can make it an enjoyable and useful part of a care plan.

The Care Act 2014 is focused on supporting people's wellbeing, and there is clear evidence that yoga can enhance wellbeing, as well as improve physical and cognitive functioning.

One of the many positive things about this book is the way in which it looks at relaxation techniques and makes them easy and accessible for people living in care homes and their families. Many of the activities outlined can also have positive benefits for the staff, and yoga is an activity that can benefit everyone and can really help us 'care for the carers'.

It is really clear when you see yoga in action that it makes a positive impact on the lives of residents and their families, but as well as seeing the results, Tania Plahay's work provides a clear evidence base of the benefits of yoga in care settings and in residential homes.

The work outlined in this book is based on a rigorous 18 months-long study into yoga and its benefits, and builds on the work that Tania has done over many years to prove that yoga does make a difference in the lives of people living in care settings, their families, friends and staff.

I have been fortunate enough to see yoga in action in care homes, and I know that it can make a real difference. I recommend every care home provider to read this book and to use it as the foundation for developing yoga within your own homes and services. Everybody in the care home will feel the benefits, and you will be able to show how your service stands out and deliver a better quality of life to your residents.

DISCLAIMER

The exercises in this book are in no way to be considered as a substitute for consultation with a medical practitioner, and should be used solely at the reader's discretion in conjunction with approved medical treatment. The author and the publisher are not responsible for any harm or damage to a person, no matter how caused, as a result of following any of the suggestions in this book.

ACKNOWLEDGEMENTS

First and foremost I would like to thank all the clients at Marlborough Court Care Home who took part in the 18-month project, 'Yoga for People Living with Dementia in Residential Care Settings'.

Working alongside the residents and the project team, learning from you all and getting your invaluable feedback was essential in developing this book and the yoga sequences within it. I would also like to thank the staff and management team for their help and support during that time.

I thank all the yoga teachers who have shared their knowledge and inspired me along my journey, including Rachel Hull, Emil Wendel, Julie Martin, Anne Smallwood, Jean Hall, Liz Lark, Simon Low, Liz Dillon and Donna Farhi.

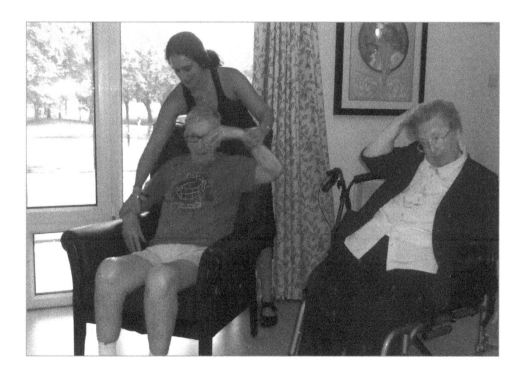

I would also like to thank the residents at Tower Bridge Care Home and in particular, Reggie and Eileen, and Maria Taylor, the activities coordinator, who first helped me set up yoga classes in residential care environments at the very start of my Yoga for Dementia journey.

Instrumental on this journey was the unflagging support of Professor Martin Green who introduced me to many people working in residential and dementia care environments. This included Maggie Candy, who is a progressive and upbeat care home manager, and has been instrumental in helping me devise and get the Yoga for Dementia project off the ground.

This book would not have been possible without the generous support of the Foundation of Nursing Studies (FoNS) and the Burdett Trust for Nursing for supporting the development, implementation and dissemination of the Yoga for Dementia Project through the Patients First programme. I would particularly like to thank Jo Odell who facilitated the programme. I learned a great deal from her about the importance of putting the patient first, and how to improve the patient's experience and my own skills in working with this group. I'd also like to thank Dr Theresa Shaw who first encouraged Maggie and me to apply for the Patients First programme.

The other project members, Hayley Mercer and Karen Cullis, made a fantastic team and brought with them a wealth of knowledge on how best to work with people living with dementia, and how to keep the sessions fun, engaging and interesting.

Andrew Houston Cummings, MBChB BSc and Registrar in General Practice, was a huge help in providing medical advice on the project.

James Heather has been a wonderful support throughout the project and the writing stage, with his active encouragement to carry on.

I would like to thank my mum, stepdad and sisters, and James' parents for their support and for encouraging me to follow my dreams!

Ken Scott, my writing coach, has been an invaluable support along the way, encouraging me to get the right words down on paper and cracking the whip to make sure I met my deadlines. He is also responsible for a lot of the photographs in the book (see www.kenscottbooks.com).

I would also like to thank Tom Mulvee, who took all the lovely photographs with the residents at Marlborough Court Care Home, and captured beautifully their engagement and enjoyment.

Rachel Menzies and Sarah Hamlin, my commissioning editors at Jessica Kingsley Publishers, have supported me throughout the writing process – thank you both.

Finally, Yin and Yang, my Spanish rescue puppies, have sat by my side throughout writing this book, keeping my legs warm and encouraging me to take regular breaks!

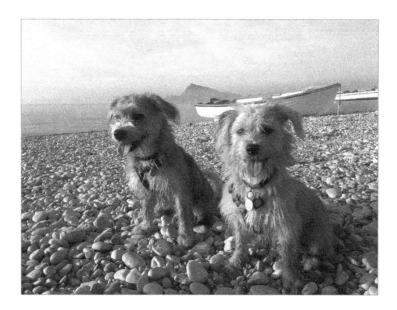

■■■ INTRODUCTION

This book aims to provide assistance to those living with dementia, their families and carers. Whilst prior experience of practising yoga would, of course, be beneficial, it is absolutely not in any way necessary to get the full benefits of the practices contained within this book. In some ways coming new to yoga at this time may be helpful, as the types of yoga employed in the sequences and the philosophy behind it may be dramatically different from most people's perception of modern yoga and any experience they may have of practising it. Many people think yoga is complicated, physically or mentally difficult, or you have to be fit and flexible to do it. This misconception is fuelled by the rise of modern western postural yoga with its images of fit, young (mainly) women with bendy bodies in contortionist-like positions.

Before reading further, try to take a moment to leave behind any doubts or concerns that you may have about any physical or mental constraints that you, or the person or people you provide care for, may have. The yoga sequences in this book have been designed, tried and tested with those living with dementia, and for those caring for them to be able to deliver. They are gentle, safe and true to the origins of yoga. Modifications are provided to allow those with increased mobility who wish to take the postures further, and also for those who are less physically able, or have any conditions or factors that mean they should not do a certain pose or exercise.

Often I hear from prospective yoga students and their families the phrases 'I won't be any good at yoga because I can't touch my toes', or 'Yoga? My mum can't do yoga, she can't even get herself dressed in the morning!' These concerns are usually based on misconceptions about yoga as being a challenging physical practice. Try to leave such preconceptions you may have about yoga behind. Yoga is a very diverse practice, and while it does contain many positions and practices that would not be suitable for those living with dementia, there are many more that are imminently suitable for those living with dementia, their loved ones and carers.

A person who practises yoga is often referred to as a 'yogi' or a 'yogini'. A yogi is someone who wants to take control of their life and feel empowered. We are all the directors of our own life movies; we choose our characters, write our scripts and make our sets. We might come from very different backgrounds, but we are united by our basic human desires to lead happy and fulfilled lives. You do not need to be a 'spiritual' person to be a yogi. Anyone can be a yogi or a yogini; all you need is the desire to find out more about yourself and others, and a desire to lead a more fulfilled life.

To set the scene, I now provide a short explanation of how I came to yoga, and how my passion led to me becoming a yoga teacher. I also explain where my interest in yoga for dementia came from.

HOW I CAME TO YOGA

I started my yoga practice when I was 18 as I was attracted by the peace and serenity I felt even after the first yoga class I took in a local gym. I loved the focus yoga gave me, and the awareness of my own body. However, back then, I thought that the main goal of yoga was to become more physically flexible, and spent my time going to mainly postural yoga classes and workshops, where teachers would guide me into more and more complex positions. I judged my progress in the practice by which bendy poses I could do and how fit and strong I felt.

Then, in my 20s, I had the opportunity to live and work in India where my paternal grandparents lived, and I spent many years there working, travelling and studying the roots of yoga. While there, I lived in yoga centres and also attended local yoga classes at community centres. What I found was mainly older people (60+) engaging in soft, gentle forms of yoga that focused on accessible positions with an emphasis on moving with awareness, addressing age-related conditions, and other forms of non-postural yoga such as the yoga of sound. This helped me understand that the essence of yoga is about ensuring it is appropriate, safe and sustainable for the students. Moving slowly with compassion and awareness is a key part of this.

As I practised more yoga and learned more about its deep history, it became an integral part of my life. Yoga was essential in helping me through periods of caring for my father who had suffered from a stroke and kidney failure whilst I was also studying full time at university. My father passed away of a heart attack when I was in my last year of university, and again, yoga helped me through the grieving process. It helped me by teaching me to stay grounded in the present moment, and not to get lost in memories. It also helped relieve the physical tension that long-term sadness brings. At my yoga classes I found myself smiling again, and also felt close to my father.

After studying yoga for over ten years with a number of teachers, I realised I wanted to spread the joys of yoga to others, and undertook training to become a yoga teacher. I was able to take a sabbatical from my government job in the UK to travel to Asia to do this. I undertook my first teacher training programme on the island of Bali, where I was fully immersed in the yogic lifestyle and practice. But it was later, while living and volunteering at a yoga centre (an ashram) specialising in gentle yoga, meditation techniques and yogic living, that I really found the path I wanted to follow. After returning to England and teaching accessible community yoga for a number of years, I knew I wanted to further my training and returned to India and enrolled in a higher level teacher training. During my yoga journey I have been lucky enough to study under some world-class teachers, and have taken what I have learned and adapted it into my own practice and teaching.

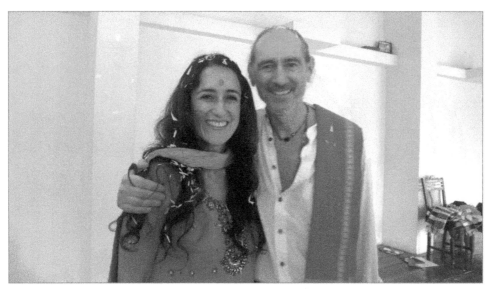

Me and my teacher, Emil Wendel

Since my advanced teacher training I have constantly sought to learn more and have specialised in a number of areas, such as training as a pregnancy and postnatal yoga teacher. Yoga is a constantly evolving field, and I believe we need to adapt the yoga we do to modern bodies and conditions. The benefits of yoga extend far beyond those gained through physical position-based classes, and I believe yoga should be offered to and available for all population groups.

When I first qualified as a teacher I began running community yoga classes in my local area to enable people with less disposable income to access it. This exposed me to all types of yoga students, from the elderly, to the complete beginner, to those already quite fit such as runners, and to those with injuries. I learned such a lot from these 'students', who I also consider to be some of my greatest teachers. They have taught me ways to adapt yoga to specific bodies and conditions, and helped me refine my teaching skills. I have also taught at various yoga retreats in Europe, which enabled me to work intensively with people over a longer period and really get to know students. Whilst I teach all ages and fitness levels, I particularly enjoy working with older people to alleviate and overcome age-related conditions.

I have also been fortunate enough to work with many people suffering from stress and anxiety through meditation and pranayama (breathing techniques) courses I have designed and led, including a popular course for the UK Houses of Parliament. Through these courses I have learned that a wide range of people from all backgrounds can benefit from simple breathing, relaxation and meditation techniques. When preparing these courses I simplified many of the more complex meditation techniques I had learned from various teachers to make them accessible to people with little or no experience in meditation. These simple techniques had a profound effect on the participants, including one student overcoming long-term anxiety issues. I found receiving such positive feedback from my courses and workshops much more satisfying than my day job.

Later, after developing and implementing my 'Yoga for Dementia' sequences in a residential care setting, I decided to focus my life entirely on yoga. I applied for and accepted voluntary redundancy from my government job and became a full-time yoga teacher. It is my passion and aim to help people access the combined benefits of the physical practice of asanas (poses), pranayama (breathing techniques) and the cognitive rejuvenation and benefits of meditation.

HOW I BECAME INVOLVED IN DEMENTIA CARE

When I was 18 and just about to start university, my father suffered from a stroke, and as he lived alone, he had to go into a nursing home for a short time before I was able to become his principal carer. I recall going to visit him in the home and seeing lots of elderly people sitting in front of the TV, not really doing anything. They were not interacting with each other or their carers, or engaging in any meaningful activities. I remember being shocked and saddened by what I saw within the nursing home, and this left a lasting impression on me.

After a few months I was able to provide care for my father at home with me. I used yoga during the time to help deal with the stresses and worries of being his principal carer, and would occasionally do yoga with him. The stroke had had a serious impact on his mobility and the things we could do together were limited. My father passed away when I was 21, which was devastating for me. However, I am eternally grateful for those last years we spent together, even though they were difficult at times for us both. He keenly felt his loss of independence and I felt the burdens of being a young carer. Although suffering from a stroke can have different impacts from dementia-related conditions, there were similarities in terms of his cognitive decline, and anger about his loss of independence. His speech was also affected, which sometimes made finding the right words and communicating difficult.

My grandmother has also been living with dementia for the last seven years. She was living a very independent life at home well into her late 80s, doing all her own gardening, cooking and baking. She passed away while I was completing this book at the age of 95. I saw the devastating effects of her illness on herself and my family. I have also witnessed the limitations it poses for her quality of life, independence and ability to make choices.

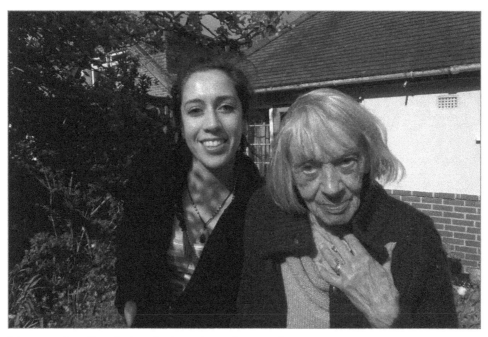

My grandmother in her beloved garden, and my sister, who did the illustrations for this book

After I had finished my first yoga teacher training and spent time living at the yoga centre (ashram), I was really touched by the idea of karma yoga, sometimes known as 'the yoga of action'. Karma yoga is a practice of giving back to your community and trying to give what you can to make the lives of those around you better. Gandhi or Mother Teresa could be considered some of the most famous karma yogis of recent times. Therefore, when I got back from my yoga teacher training, I wanted to serve my local community, and also help spread the simple and wonderful yoga techniques to a wider audience. I became involved at my local nursing home in running simple chair-based yoga sessions once a week. Working with these residents I devised some early sequences that the residents found both engaging and relaxing. After working with this group for a few months I began to notice the benefits of the yoga for these elderly residents, including those living with dementia.

Some of those I worked with were angry, and this both challenged but also improved my teaching practice, and my understanding of the stresses carers and family members are under. Many of the residents did not get involved in any other activities on offer, but took part in the yoga, and their carers reported improvements in their mood as well as physical benefits such as an increased range of motion. I worked with residents with a number of medical conditions and of different ages up to the age of 96. I still remember the joy I saw on their faces as they did the simple yoga exercises, and their pleasure in learning new skills. People grow from learning new skills, and I strongly believe that when we stop learning, we stop fully living. More and more, through working with the older generations, I have been surprised at how open they are to learning new things. This inspired me to have a vision of spreading simple yoga exercises to more nursing homes, and benefiting those living with dementia and other supposedly 'limiting' conditions.

EILEEN'S STORY

Eileen was one of the first students I worked with in a residential care setting. She was wheelchair-bound and had painful and limiting swelling of her joints. Eileen did not join in any of the other activities within the home, and did not socialise with other residents. The weekly yoga classes I was running at the time gave her welcome relief from her painful swelling, and she would remember and practise the sequences during the week in the comfort of her own room. Although quite shy, Eileen found much joy in the singing practices we would do together with the group.

Through working with my local nursing home I was lucky to meet Professor Martin Green, who is Chief Executive of Care England (the umbrella body for independent care homes). He introduced me to a dynamic care home manager who was interested in offering her residents a more holistic approach to their care. Together, we applied for and succeeded in winning grant funding for a competitive programme called Patients First, run by the Foundation of Nursing Studies (FoNS) and the Burdett Trust for Nursing. This programme is designed to promote innovation in the way nursing care is delivered and to improve the patient's experience. The project I designed and implemented developed and tested yoga for people in residential care with a particular focus on those living with dementia. It involved a multidisciplinary team of experts, and drew on advice and training from a wide range of people including medical research professionals. I developed many of the sequences contained within this book as part of this project.

The formal project trial period was completed in November 2014. The results of the project showed that the yoga sequences had had a positive physical and mental effect on the residents. In addition, through my own experience as a carer and working on this project, I have seen first hand how yoga can improve the caring experience by providing meaningful, calming, simple and beneficial activities. This, and the huge need for ways of improving the lives of those living with dementia, has inspired me to take my research and teaching in this field further. I am now working on rolling this programme out at a large number of care homes. Further information on the project can be found on my website (see www.yoga4dementia.com).

WHO THE BOOK IS AIMED AT

This book is aimed at people who have had an early diagnosis of dementia, or who have a family history of dementia and are worried about possible signs of cognitive impairment. The exercises and practices in this book will help you live more in the moment, and improve your day-to-day health and wellbeing.

While the book is also intended for family and professional caregivers, and will give you the skills to introduce your clients to some simple and effective yoga techniques, you are also highly likely to benefit from these techniques yourself.

The book also provides a useful general introduction to accessible and gentle yoga, and can be used as a general introductory text for people wanting to start yoga in later life. It is also very beneficial for those living with injuries.

HOW TO USE THE BOOK

This book provides a wealth of resources for a variety of readers. It might be that you have just been diagnosed with Alzheimer's or another form of dementia, and are seeking practices that will help you stay well for longer and will stimulate your mind. It might be that you have a family member with dementia and are looking for appropriate and meaningful activities to do together. You might be a yoga teacher looking to run classes for those living with dementia.

When reading this book I recommend a number of approaches. If you are completely new to yoga, and do not know much about dementia, you could read this book straight through. Alternatively, you might want to skip to a section that interests you most, for example, one on softer and more relaxing practices. Or maybe one of the anger management practices. As emphasised throughout the book, yoga is something you need to experience for yourself, so please do take time out to do the exercises described. A number of video resources are also available for readers of this book, and they can be accessed at www.jkp.com/voucher using the code PLAHAYYOGA.

One of the key things we should do as we embark on this yoga journey is to buy a small notebook. This should be used to keep track of the exercises we have practised, and the effects of these. If we, ourselves, are living with dementia, this can provide a great record of which things we have practised, and how they made us feel. If you are working with people with later stages of dementia, the notebook can provide a helpful document of your own journey as you learn to introduce these practices to others. You can also record which exercises worked best with the person or people you care for, and the effects on them.

If you are thinking of starting a yoga practice yourself, and have any pre-existing conditions or other concerns, it is important to talk to your doctor about your intention to start a yoga practice. You might like to show your doctor this book, or your notebook so that they can see that the practices contained in it are suitable for you.

NAME	INFO
Easy exercise	This symbol indicates very simple exercises that can be done by anyone. If you are new to yoga or living with the later stages of dementia these are good exercises to start with.
Medium exercise	This symbol indicates slightly more complex exercises which are good once you have mastered some of the easy exercises.
Complex exercise	This symbol indicates more challenging exercises which are good to simulate your mind and body.
Partner exercise	This symbol indicates an exercise which is best to do with a partner.
Caring for the carer exercise	This symbol indicates exercises which are specifically good for those caring for someone living with dementia.
Physical exercises and sequences	This symbol indicates physical exercises which can help older adults reach exercise targets.
Meditation and Guided Relaxation and exercises for promoting better sleep	This symbol indicates meditation and guided relaxation, and those exercises that are calming/good for sleep.
Rescue remedy for times of stress and anxiety	This symbol indicates exercises that are particularly good for times of stress, anger and anxiety.
Quick exercises	This symbol indicates quick 5–15. minute exercises.
Longer sequences/ practices	This symbol indicates longer practices and sequences.
Audio	This symbol indicates that there is an accompanying audio file.
Video	This symbol indicates that there is an accompanying video file.

CHAPTER 1

WHAT IS YOGA?

So you have heard about how yoga has helped me throughout my life, and how beneficial it can be for those living with dementia. But what is yoga? Is it about touching your toes and contorting your body into difficult pretzel-like shapes? Whilst yoga does contain some emphasis on physical positions (known as asanas), this is merely a small part of a wider body of yoga.

There are many definitions of yoga, and these can range from 'union of mind, body and spirit', 'balance' to the 'cessations of turmoil in the mind'. The word *yoga* comes from the ancient Indian language Sanskrit word *yuj*, which means 'yoke': this is the device used to attach a bull to a cart, and embodies the idea of joining something together. In its essence it derives from the idea of creating a union of the brain and the body, the self and others, and the mind and spirit. Yoga can also be described as achieving a state of oneness, but it is often used to describe the practices we do to try and attain this state.

Although yoga has its roots in ancient India, it is a secular practice, and you do not have to be a Hindu, Buddhist or from any other religion to practise it. Some yoga practices might encourage a sense of surrender to a higher being or power, but, for example, if you are a Christian, this higher power could be Christ, or if you are a Muslim, it could be Allah, or any other personal god or belief system, so if mountains inspire you, your personal higher power could be the power of nature.

In simple terms, yoga is a holistic practice that unites mind, body and breath. There are many forms, but 'doing yoga' often involves some simple physical exercises called *asanas* (or positions). The key original yoga texts (see below) address asanas very briefly, and state that you should aim to attain a steady and comfortable position. Although these postures have become more and more complex, the origins of yoga show that they should be simple but done with awareness, steadiness and ease. They will also often have physical benefits; for example, gentle backbends help to open the heart and lung area and stimulate the body, whereas twists help to stimulate the digestive system.

These positions are often combined with other aspects of yoga. For example, the yamas and niyamas are inward and outward 'codes' of conduct. These include elements such as contentment (santosha) and non-violence (ahimsa). Santosha is about trying to be content with what we have in our lives, which can be useful for coming to terms with the changes ageing and dementia bring. Ahimsa is the practice of non-violence. It is about being non-violent to ourselves in our physical practice and thoughts, as well as being non-violent to others. We explore these codes of conduct and how they can be helpful later in the book (see 'Eight limbs of yoga' on page 46, Chapter 3).

Practising yoga might also involve simple breathing exercises known as *pranayama* that help to improve the functioning of the lungs, bring more energy and vitality to the body, and promote calmness in times of stress or anxiety. Often when we are mentally tense we also tense our bodies. We might hold this stress in our shoulders, or clench our jaws, or hold our abdomen in. This creates energy blockages in the body. In yoga it is believed that when energy is blocked, this creates tension and ill health. In a way, energy blockages can be compared to when our arteries become blocked by a build-up of fat, or when neurons get blocked by plaque. Blood, or electrical energy, does not flow as well and we will get 'bottlenecks' with in the physical pathways of the body. Newcomers to yoga often find that when we release physical tension, we also release mental tension, and so they often feel a sense of relief after classes.

Yoga practice might also include some *guided relaxations or meditation*. There is more and more knowledge about the benefits of meditation and in particular, its role in reducing stress and anxiety. I have seen first hand how clients from all walks of life and all ages benefit from guided relaxations. This is particularly beneficial for those living with dementia, as people find being gently guided by the human voice helps them relax.

Yoga can also involve the use of *mantras*. A mantra is a sacred sound, syllable, prayer or phrase that is repeated. The practice is common in many religions such as Hinduism, Buddhism, Christianity, Jainism and Sikhism, but, as explained later, in Chapter 13, it is not necessary to be religious to practise mantras. There are a number of ways that mantras are said to work. In yoga it is believed that all the external impressions of the world are known as samskaras, and that these can shape our brains and thought patterns, including negative thoughts. Therefore, if we replace negative thoughts with positive mantras, this helps to reshape our thought patterns. The power of suggestion and belief is high, as seen by the famous 'placebo' effect, whereby in drug trials, even those patients given the dummy drug show signs of improvement if they believe they are given the right drug. A mantra can also work in this way. It is also believed that the 'sounds' of the mantra create an internal vibration that has a positive effect on the cells and internal structure of the body. Scientists have supported this theory, and a number of papers show that sound has a direct and indirect effect on cells and the growth of microbes (e.g. Gu, Zhang and Wu 2016).

Modern yoga also draws from recently developed secular *mindfulness practices*. These have been tried and tested and seen to be effective in reducing stress. For example, mindfulness-based stress reduction courses have been shown to help dramatically reduce pain, and improve people's ability to relax (Chiesa and Serretti 2009). During a yoga class a teacher may encourage the student to remain focused in the present, and this is a key factor in ensuring the practice remains safe.

There are many *different types of yoga*; for example, karma yoga is known as the 'yoga of action'. This may involve following a calling, caring for a loved one or helping those in need. It is about taking action without expectations of rewards. Bhakti yoga is a 'yoga of devotion'; it often means following a path of loving devotion, and may involve singing devotional songs. Nada yoga, or the 'yoga of sound', uses singing and chanting to help with healing.

In summary, there are many practices that might make up a 'yoga class or session', and yoga might also refer as much to a state of being or attitude as performing a specific task or exercise. Further details of types of poses or practices can be found in the sequences section of this book (Chapters 4 and 8–14).

THE ORIGINS OF YOGA

So, you might be wondering, where did this practice of yoga come from, how old is it and who developed it?

The true origins of yoga are difficult to pinpoint exactly. Prior to written records, teachings on yoga would have been passed down by oral tradition from a teacher (sometimes known as a guru, which means dispeller of darkness) to a student. Even when texts were put 'down on paper', the 'paper' was fragile palm leaves that quickly became damaged, if not lost entirely. While some historians cite the beginnings of yoga as far back as 10,000 years ago, ancient Indian seals like the one shown on the next page show figures in what clearly look like yoga positions, and these date from 3500 and 1900 BCE. However, it was not until 2000 years ago that the various ideas came together and were put down in one place.

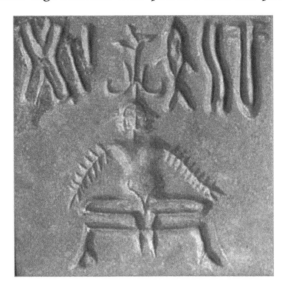

At some point between 200 BCE and 200 CE Patanjali's Yoga Sutras, a collection of 195 short verses, were transcribed. Patanjali was considered to be a Rishi (Indian Sage), and he is often considered the father of yoga; he was also the author of a number of other texts, for example, on grammar and Ayurveda (yoga's sister science, which is sometimes called the science of life). These texts were written in Sanskrit, an ancient Indian language.

The Yoga Sutras contain information about what yoga is and how to practise it. They describe eight limbs (or parts) of yoga – our inward and outward conduct, physical positions, breathing exercises, withdrawing the senses, focus, meditation and achieving bliss (see 'Eight limbs of yoga' on page 44, Chapter 3). The goal of yoga was about creating balance in life, getting to know oneself better, contentment, finding fulfilment and learning to be the best person we can be. There are many paths to achieving this state of 'yoga', for example, karma yoga (the yoga of action), bhakti yoga (the yoga of loving devotion) and raja yoga (meditation and knowledge).

Yoga continued to be practised in the sub-continent, and over time it became influenced by other 'strands' of thought and knowledge. For example, Tibetan monks practised a form of yoga linked to Tibetan medicine, and many of the meditation techniques we practise in modern yoga may have their origins in Buddhism. Yoga was also influenced by the philosophy of non-harming from the Jains (another religion that was founded in India around the same time as Buddhism), and non-attachment from wandering sadhus or holy men who would perform extreme physical feats to test their mental and physical strength.

THE ARRIVAL OF YOGA IN THE WEST

Yoga became popular in the west in the 1960s and 1970s through influential teachers such as B.K.S. Iyengar and Swami Paramahansa Yogananda. It was further popularised by pop groups such as the Beatles, who famously practised transcendental meditation techniques with a renowned guru, Maharishi Mahesh Yogi, in Rishikesh, India. In the heady days of the 1960s, yoga was seen as groovy, mysterious and fashionable.

Since the beginning of the 21st century there has been a huge increase in the number of people practising yoga in the west. Predictably, the rise of modern yoga has also been accompanied by a huge rise in the 'business of yoga' or yoga merchandising such as yoga equipment and clothing. Any business is accompanied by the idea of selling, and to fuel this we have seen a rise in 'spiritual materialism' or the idea of 'collecting' spiritual experiences or practices. In relation to this, many teachers have made yoga practices more complex and physically difficult as they try to 'sell' more experiences and practices or create 'unique' products.

Many yoga schools and practitioners still practise and teach forms of yoga that are more focused on physical development than on mental growth, with people transitioning to practising yoga from aerobics, Pilates and other gym-based activities. People in western societies generally have fast-paced lives, high-pressure jobs and suffer from stress. Time set aside for yoga classes is usually brief, and there is an expectation for a maximum return on their investment of time and energy. This approach has led to a massive explosion in recent years of fitness-based yoga classes, which are sometimes led by personal trainers with scant yoga qualifications, or by yoga teachers whose main aim is to improve the physical body. You may have heard of some of these yoga styles being branded as 'power yoga' or other similar adjectives. Many athletes also use yoga in combination with weight training to reduce injuries. Others perform yoga in hot environments akin to a sauna, intending to lose weight and cleanse by sweating heavily. There is some truth that a warm environment can relax muscles, allowing easier stretching, but this also puts people at risk of over-stretching ligaments, muscles and joints beyond what they would normally be able to achieve without being put off by pain, and this can result in serious injuries.

These high-energy yoga classes, weight loss-focused techniques and fitness-fuelled styles of teaching definitely have their place, and in general, I am always pleased to see the global growth of yoga. However, in some cases, they can result in injury that goes against one of the principles of yoga, which is ahimsa, or 'non-harming'. These styles are also very different from the origins of yoga and the practices I teach and follow. I believe in an inclusive understanding of yoga, as a gentle and accepting practice that balances mind and body, and that can be applied throughout life.

THE BENEFITS OF YOGA

In the early days of yoga people would have experienced its physical and mental benefits, and this is probably one of the reasons for its spread and continued evolution. Yoga also emerged in a time of high culture in ancient India when much was known about the body. Specific systems of ancient medicine and healing were used, including the popular science of Ayurveda that is still used today. Medicine and healing would have happened on a local level. However, it was not until the start of 'western medicine' that the benefits of yoga needed to be 'scientifically' proven in strict research trials.

In the early 1920s Swami Kuvalayanada founded the Kaivalyadham Health and Yoga Research Centre and Shri Yogendraji founded the Yoga Institute, which started scientific research into the effects of yoga postures and breathing exercises. These, and other Indian yoga institutions and research centres, have continued to grow and research the benefits of yoga, including the well-known Yoga Research Foundation run by the Bihar School of Yoga. More recently in the west we have seen a growth in the emerging field of 'yoga therapy'. In contrast to fitness-orientated group classes, this is where a yoga therapist will work directly with a client, or a group of clients, with specific issues. As yoga has spread and gained more interest from the scientific community, more and more verified research has been done on the medical benefits of yoga, for example, for back pain, or stress and anxiety.

In 2007 Dr Timothy McCall published a book called *Yoga as Medicine*, which provides yoga prescriptions and case studies for a number of medical conditions. The introduction to this book summarised a number of research papers and studies, and showed that yoga can improve a vast range of common conditions including anxiety, asthma, back pain, balance problems, bladder dysfunction, dementia, depression, diabetes, emphysema, gait (walking) problems, heart disease, high blood pressure, insomnia, irritable bowel syndrome, neck pain, osteoarthritis, osteoporosis, rehabilitation and post-operative recovery, rheumatoid arthritis, sinusitis, stress incontinence and stroke.

In 2016 a team at the University of California and Los Angeles (UCLA) found that yoga helped reduce pre-Alzheimer's cognitive impairment (Eyre *et al.* 2016). Earlier, in 2012, dru yoga was shown to reduce perceived stress and back pain at work (Hartfiel *et al.* 2012). Furthermore, many studies have also shown that practices such as yoga and meditation help to turn on the relaxation response (RR) that is said to counter the stresses of everyday life. People who regularly practise RR techniques show physiological changes including decreased oxygen consumption, reduced blood pressure, heart and respiration rate, and alterations in the brain. A 2008 study also found altered gene expression in specific functional groups, which suggests a greater capacity to respond to oxidative stress and associated cellular damage (Dusek *et al.* 2008).

HOW YOGA WORKS

- Yoga can change the subtle hormonal balances in the body and stimulate the production of 'rest and restore' and feel-good hormones such as endorphins, and reduce stress hormones such as cortisol and adrenaline.

- Yoga helps to stimulate and stretch and tone the whole body. This increases the movement of muscles and has positive effects on the circulatory system.

- On a physical level yoga improves breathing by making the breath slower, deeper and more effective, thereby increasing the flow of oxygen to muscles and organs and removing waste products, aiding recovery and healing.

- Breathing slowly and deeply is said to help promote a sense of calm, relaxation and wellbeing. Breath work also raises the level of serotonin and lowers the levels of monoamine oxidase that feature in depression, which can be a common side effect of dementia.

- Some yoga poses such as backbends (which can be performed on a chair) are energising, and some poses are relaxing. This combination of physical and mental stimulation and relaxation is beneficial for physical and mental health.

- Yoga, through coordinated movement, also helps to stimulate under-used nerve pathways in the brain, and can therefore help the mind as well as the body.

- Yoga, and particularly the guided relaxations, can help people move into an internal still place, where they are not focused on their own anxiety.

- Yoga can also help with anger management. For example, particular postures such as 'lion's breath' (see page 188), or using sound-based yoga, are a great way to release the physical restlessness in the body and mind that comes with anger.

- Yoga involves periods of being very calm and focused on the present moment. This can help those living with dementia and those supporting them come to terms with the changes that are happening to them through accepting the present and not trying to recreate the past, or becoming too focused on regrets.

- Meditation is also important for the mind, and can help those living with dementia find peace and come to terms with the changes in their lives in a calm way, including preparing for the later stages of life.

Later in this book we explore further how yoga can help specifically with those living with various stages of dementia.

YOGA IN THIS BOOK

- It is my intention to demystify yoga practices and to show that there are *suitable and appropriate yoga sequences* for people living with all stages of dementia. These simple sessions can be delivered by families, carers, activities coordinators or others based in residential care environments, and provide meaningful, fun and calming practices to do together.

- The yoga in this book is firmly rooted in the classical *yoga philosophy*. It combines various aspects of yoga and is based on the principles of ahimsa (non-harming) and karma yoga. This book is my karma yoga or yoga of service for those living with dementia, their families and carers.

- I have focused on bringing a *range of yogic techniques* together from both the traditional schools of hatha yoga to more modern schools such as vinyasa, which emphasises flowing and graceful movements that move with the breath (for more about the different types of yoga, see Chapter 2). This book includes guided meditations, visualisations, breathing techniques, hand gestures and sound practices from a range of traditions. These techniques have been tested over a period of many years, and I have seen first hand the benefits these have brought to many people from different backgrounds. Although the techniques in this book are largely aimed at those living with dementia, my research has shown that they also have many positive benefits for their families and carers too.

- The sequences begin with *gentle physical movements* that help to get the student used to moving more. These movements provide physical exercise for the whole body, and in particular, to often neglected muscle groups in older people. Some of the exercises help to develop mobility, confidence, coordination and balance. New movements themselves help to activate the brain. Sound is incorporated into some movements as additional stimulus.

- Specific *breathing techniques* are also taught and employed throughout the sequences, which have a variety of physical and mental benefits. For example, increasing oxygen to the muscles and the brain helps to promote a restful and calm state. A variety of guided meditation techniques are used throughout the book that can be highly beneficial in helping clients and their carers deal with stress and anxiety.

It is my sincere hope that these simple and effective yoga-based practices outlined in this book bring more joy and peace into the lives of those living with dementia.

CONCLUSION

In this chapter we have explored some of the many definitions of yoga, and the fact that yoga refers to a diverse set of different practices. Yoga is not a religion and can be practiced by people of all faiths, or none. We also briefly touched on the origins of yoga, this intends to set the scene for the book, rather than be an exhaustive guide to all the roots of yoga. Yoga has many paths and methods and this chapter has shown that there are yoga practices that can benefit us all. This chapter also briefly touches on how yoga works and brings benefits to those who practice. Yoga does not have to be complex and difficult; all we need to do is set aside a small amount of time each week to practice. Whenever we embark on any new actively or journey it is good to be clear about our intentions. Your intention for reading this book might be to find ways of being more in the moment, or improving your day-to-day wellbeing. The chapter concludes with my intensions for this book and my sincere hope that you, your loved ones, and/or those that you care for can benefit from the wide-ranging practices within this book. Why not take a moment to write your intention now in your notebook?

CHAPTER 2

TYPES OF YOGA

As explained in Chapter 1, yoga has had a huge growth since the beginning of the 21st century. In fact, in the US it is currently one of the fastest growing forms of 'exercise'. With this growth yoga has developed and evolved from the traditional practices done in India. In general this evolution has brought a focus on more dynamic asana-based practices (physical positions), which emphasise difficult positions and are more suitable for young and physically fit practitioners. Often with this type of yoga comes a competitive and commercial edge, with classes being quite expensive and a focus on expensive yoga 'gear' such as clothing, mats etc. I recently heard about a case in London where a well-known yoga studio made all of its instructors reapply for their jobs. One of the key criteria for getting a post was the number of social media followers they had. Often such teachers will post thousands of pictures of themselves doing 'difficult' positions in a bid to improve their 'online' presence.

Of course, marketing is a necessary part of modern society and getting information to the right people. However, I believe that a teacher should be rated on their ability to teach, rather than what they look like doing a yoga pose, and how many Instagram followers they have. My key point is that this commercialisation has emphasised the difficult parts of yoga, and you might have seen such pictures and thought that yoga is not suitable for you or those you might care for. However, this type of asana-focused yoga is only the superficial tip of a large iceberg of simple, deep and satisfying practices that you do not need to be a size 8 and under the age of 25 to practise.

Sometimes people tell me that they have tried yoga and do not like it. When I encounter someone like this I always recommend that they try another teacher or another style of yoga. There are so many types and ranges of different practices I am convinced that there are types of yoga to suit every type of person.

When you start practising yoga, or teaching it to your loved one or clients, I am sure your friends and relatives will be interested in what you are doing and you might get asked what type of yoga you are practising and/or leading. Alternatively, if you have a mild cognitive impairment (MCI) or are a carer/family member who is just starting to try yoga, it is highly likely that you will experience the benefits for yourself and want to explore yoga further. Therefore, in what follows I have given a brief explanation of some of the different 'types' of yoga that are around today. If asked, the yoga practices in this book provide a synthesis of a variety of types.

I introduce you here to some of the key styles, as I want to ensure that you are equipped with the tools and knowledge to choose a relevant style of yoga for you to practise or to recommend to a friend, family member or colleague. However, there is no need for you to explore other classes further at the moment, as this book has adapted some of the best and most appropriate exercises from the key schools of yoga, combining these into an accessible format. In my own training and study of yoga philosophy, yoga is about unity, not division, and choosing the most appropriate exercises for your body. Therefore it is very important to be able to access and choose the most appropriate yoga exercises for you or the person you are caring for. If you would like to experience going to a class, or want to further your knowledge, please do check out the 'Further Reading and Resources' section at the end of this book, or one of the styles recommended below.

TRADITIONAL STYLES OF YOGA

Traditional styles of yoga are generally those that follow classical Indian yoga texts. They tend to emphasise yoga as a rounded practice that goes beyond a narrow focus on physical positions.

Hatha yoga

Hatha yoga is a combination of classical yoga asanas (physical positions) and pranayama (breath work). The word 'ha-tha' means to exert force, and this type of yoga requires some physical effort in completing the physical asanas and pranayama. The sequences of the positions are designed to help align your skin, muscles and bones. The positions are also aimed at opening the energy channels of the body – especially the spine, which is considered the body's main information 'super-highway'. Hatha is also often translated as *ha*, meaning 'sun', and *tha*, meaning 'moon'. This refers to the balance of the different energies within us all, in particular, the masculine energy – active, hot, sun – and the feminine energy – receptive, cool, moon. Hatha yoga is often used to describe gentle, physical yoga, a series of non-flowing static poses.

Sivananda yoga

Swami Sivananda was one of the key well-known yogis who popularised yoga in the west. In his early life he served as a physician for the British Army. In the 1930s and 1940s Sivananda founded a number of prominent yoga schools such as the Divine Life Society, and is the author of over 200 books on yoga and other subjects. Sivananda yoga is very popular today, and is practised throughout the world.

Sivananda yoga is a balanced form of yoga that has five key parts:

1. Exercise, in particular, the daily practice of sun salutations and 12 core positions.

2. Breathing, in particular, full yogic breath (see 'Three-part breath' on page 61, Chapter 4) and alternate nostril breathing (or nadi shodhana) (see page 208, Chapter 11).

3. Relaxing, including physical, mental and spiritual relaxing.

4. Diet, including mainly whole foods.

5. Positive mental attitude and meditation.

Satyananda yoga

Swami Sivananda had many prominent disciples who went on to found their own yoga schools including Satyananda. Satyananda is one of my personal favourite schools of traditional yoga. Satyananda Saraswati founded the Bihar School of Yoga, which has been responsible for spreading many of the ancient yoga techniques through its accessible yoga publications, some of which are recommended in the 'Further Reading and Resources' section. Satyananda yoga again is a balanced form of yoga, which incorporates the whole body.

Bhakti yoga

Bhakti yoga is concerned with feelings of unity with a divine super soul or form. *Bhakti* is a Sanskrit term that signifies an attitude of devotion to a personal 'god'. It is often considered to be the easiest way for ordinary people to attain a spiritually liberated state, because although it is a form of yoga, its practice is not as rigorous as many other yogic methods. For more bhakti yoga practices, see Chapter 13.

Kundalini yoga

Kundalini yoga is a physically and mentally challenging practice that is very different from what you might expect of a 'typical' yoga class. It aims to awaken the dormant energy that is said to lie at the base of your spine. When practising kundalini yoga you will work on a variety of kriyas (physical or mental exercises), which are sometimes combined with breath work, chanting, singing and meditation. A well-known kriya practice is kirtan kriya (singing practice) outlined on page 159 in Chapter 9. The aim of kundalini yoga is to unleash our internal energy and to bring ourselves to a higher level of awareness. It goes beyond some yoga practices by having a greater focus on our internal energy.

There are many other traditional schools of yoga that emphasise a balance of different yoga practices, and encourage the adoption of a yogic lifestyle. These forms are often simple and accessible, and suitable for people from all walks of life.

MODERN YOGA STYLES

As yoga has developed and increased in popularity, many different styles have developed. These might involve specific sequences or approaches or different aspects of focus. For example, jivamukti yoga includes chanting in each class, and has an emphasis on inverted poses. Dharma yoga emphasises good health, a clear mind and a kind heart. Anusara yoga focuses on opening the heart.

Iyengar yoga

B.K.S. Iyengar was a hugely influential teacher who did a great deal to popularise yoga in the west. He was a student of Tirumalai Krishnama-charya, who is considered the 'father of modern yoga'. As a sickly child

Iyengar was taught yoga by Krishnamacharya, and used it to develop his strength and stamina. He wrote one of the seminal texts on yoga, *Light on Yoga* (which contains detailed instructions on some of the key positions), as well as other books on yoga philosophy and breathing. Iyengar yoga uses blocks and belts and other 'props' to ensure correct yoga positions. It also focuses on long hold positions. This form of yoga is suitable for those with injuries, as it emphasises good alignment and safe and sustainable positions. It was one of the first types of yoga I studied, and I was drawn to its preciseness and focus on alignment.

Ashtanga vinyasa yoga

K. Pattabhi Jois, another one of Krishnamacharya's disciples, developed ashtanga vinyasa yoga. This is a challenging and dynamic form of yoga that I would say is generally best suited to those who are young and relatively fit. It consists of six series of poses that get progressively harder. Between each pose there is a sequence of movements known as a vinyasa.

Vinyasa yoga

Vinyasa yoga is a modern form of yoga that has been developed from a blend of ashtanga yoga and other forms. It involves adapted sequences of flowing poses that link together. It aims to take the body through a range of movements, and can range from being quite fast to more slow-paced. I studied vinyasa yoga, and some of the sequences in this book take a vinyasa-like approach, which emphasises moving gradually into positions and using the body's natural range of movements.

Yin and restorative yoga

Yin and restorative yoga are both styles that emphasise holding positions for a long period. Yin is more focused on poses that help target deeper connective tissues, whilst restorative yoga is more about poses that focus on letting go and using the force of gravity to help relax the body. Often restorative yoga will involve the use of props, such as a pillow, to help you relax completely. Restorative yoga helps to activate the parasympathetic nervous system (PNS) (for more about this, see 'Key ways in which yoga works' on page 88, Chapter 5). Restorative yoga is great for those who have a hard time slowing down; it can also be wonderful if you are having trouble sleeping, or are suffering from stress or anxiety. It is particularly beneficial for carers who are on their feet a lot, and who need to unwind. Try some restorative yoga poses from Chapter 4.

YOGA THERAPY

Yoga therapy is a growing field of yoga focusing specifically on how yoga can heal and help with many diseases. It can both help prevent diseases and also help with recovery times. There is now a professional body for yoga therapy, and more and more studies are being done on the benefits of yoga. The Kaivalyadharma Health and Yoga Research Centre, which is in India, is one of the oldest yoga therapy schools. The International Yoga Therapy Association is a newer organisation that has its headquarters in the USA. This body publishes a journal and also has regular conferences.

CONCLUSION

In this chapter I have emphasised that yoga is for everybody, and it really does not matter what size, shape, fitness level or age you are! There are practices within this book that you can safely start right now. We have explored some of the main schools or branches of yoga, including traditional and modern yoga. Of course this is not an exhaustive list and there are many more schools and types of yoga I don't have room in the book to include. Also for ease I have simplified the descriptions of the types of yoga. However I hope this chapter has piqued your interest into different types of yoga, and encouraged you to learn more. I finish by introducing the field of yoga therapy and if you are interested more in this topic I'd highly recommend the *Yoga as Medicine* (McCall 2007) book in the recommended reading and resources section.

CHAPTER 3

YOGA PHILOSOPHY AND PRINCIPLES

In this chapter we explore some yoga philosophy and principles, including some exercises we can do together. Like modern life, yoga has many layers, and yoga poses can range from the complex to the very simple. The fact that yoga is simple enough to be experienced by beginners, but also contains many levels, means that once you have learned some of the basic principles, you can delve deeper into the practices and learn more.

Patanjali, who is considered to be the father of yoga, and was said to live in the 2nd century BC (although the practice of yoga is thought to be much older), codified some of the basic principles of yoga. He categorised yoga into eight limbs (parts or branches). We now explore these limbs and some simple introductory exercises. I recommend that you read this section slowly and use your notebook to write down some of your reactions to these exercises, or make notes of those you would like to try.

EIGHT LIMBS OF YOGA

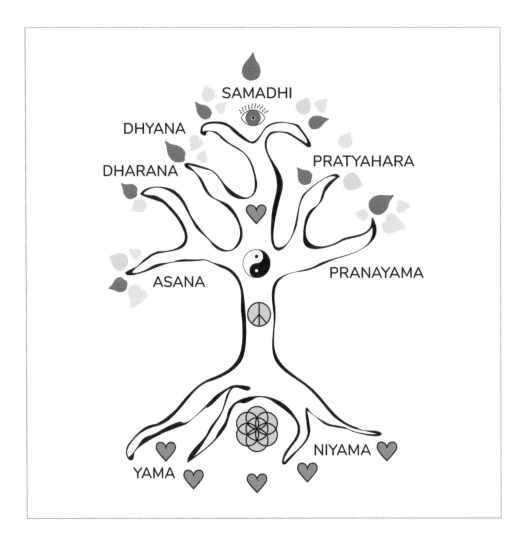

1. Yamas

The first part of yoga is about how we treat others in life and our outward conduct in the world. In yoga terms these are called *yamas*, and put simply, this is about treating others how we would like to be treated ourselves. There are five aspects of the yamas.

Ahimsa, or non-violence. Ahimsa is about not hurting ourself or others. It is about being tolerant to other people's differences. Sometimes when we think about violence we might primarily think about physical violence, but much violence in the world starts with mental violence. For example, this can occur when we think violent, non-tolerant or judgemental thoughts about ourselves and others. In Chapter 10 I have provided an exercise to explore our understanding of violence and how to reduce these thoughts ('Anger meditation' page 176).

Satya, or truthfulness. This yama is about not aiming to deceive ourselves or others, and conveying what we know to be truthful. So, for example, when we have been diagnosed with dementia we might deceive our families or ourselves about our diagnosis as we are scared about the disease's progression or our family's reaction to it. We might lie to those around us 'to be nice', or for some other reason we tell ourselves. However, if we do not speak truthfully, it often comes out later to haunt us. Most lies, even small ones, are based on fear, so we might lie to someone about the reason we were late as we are scared they will think less of us if we tell the truth. Although admitting to being scared can make us vulnerable, there is nothing wrong with being vulnerable, and often admitting we are frightened allows others around us to open up and be more truthful.

In this exercise we can explore what truthfulness means for us. It is useful for those who are living with early stages of dementia, and can also be useful for carers and family members.

  ## TRUTHFULNESS EXERCISE

Find a quiet place and make sure you have a sheet of blank paper and a pen. Set a timer for 12 minutes. Then start writing about anything you have not been honest about with yourself or with others. It could be about your diagnosis of dementia, or the person you are caring for. It could be about personal regrets you have had, but that you have kept deep inside and never discussed with others. See if you can use the time fully, even if you use it more for thinking than writing. Once you have finished writing, take a moment to reflect on the things you have written, and then rip your paper to tiny shreds. Take a moment to see if you feel any lighter having let go of those things.

Asteya, or non-stealing. Asteya is about not taking what is not given. So, whilst it can be related to physically stealing, it can also be related to taking someone's ideas without acknowledging the source, or wanting to live someone else's life. We can also 'steal' time from people by being late, we 'steal' quiet from people by always talking, or 'steal' attention from someone by always interrupting them, or finishing their sentences for them. This tends to happen a lot in mid-stage dementia when a carer or family member will often answer for the person living with dementia. If this happens with you, try to give someone more time to describe their feelings or experiences in their own words. If they cannot use words, see if you can just sit with them without talking, but watch their facial expressions.

Brahmacharya, or preserving vital energy. Brahmacharya is often related to the conserving of sexual energy, and treating each other as human beings rather than as sexual objects, but it can also be about not wasting energy. So, for example, we can waste our energy through the pursuing of sex to gratify our own ego, but we can also waste it through meaningless gossip about other people. Next time you are going to tell a story or recount an event, take a breath and think about the point of telling the story. Is it merely to make yourself look good or popular, or to shock or amuse? Does it look down on the person or situation the story is about? If this is the case, maybe reconsider telling it. This way we can avoid negative energy. Eleanor Roosevelt is credited with saying, 'Great minds discuss ideas; average minds discuss events; small minds discuss people.' Of course, everyone occasionally talks about other people, but see if you can observe what the main topics of your conversations are about, and if they tend to be mostly gossip, or complaining about others, see if you can spend more time listening. We can learn a lot from listening.

Aparigraha, or non-grasping. Aparigraha can be roughly translated as having an absence of greed. Greed can be physical, for example, for food, or material, for things like clothing; however, it can also be for experiences. Greed is often self-serving, and comes from the idea of wanting more and more. When someone has dementia, often in the early stages they become worried about losing things and may get obsessive about this. It is also common for someone to become obsessive about food. Therefore, in the early stages of dementia, it can be beneficial to practise non-hoarding or greed.

Think, for example, about letting go of something that does not serve you. On a practical level this could mean giving away some of your possessions, or helping someone you are caring for give things away gradually. In India, many people, once they reach a certain age, devote their lives to spiritual matters, and as part of this they will give away the majority of their possessions so they can be unburdened by them. The 'first people' (Native Americans) in Canada and the US also have 'give away' ceremonies where they donate many of their loved possessions so someone else can benefit from them.

As part of you committing to a regular yoga practice, or helping someone commit to theirs, why not ceremonially give away something to make space for the new practices in your life? This could be a piece of furniture or something in your room.

2. Niyamas

The next limb of yoga is the niyamas. The niyamas are about our personal discipline and how we look after ourselves. They relate both to our physical body, and also to our mental thoughts.

Sauca, or cleanliness. This is to do with external cleanliness, and also internal cleanliness. For example, it can include thinking good thoughts, staying positive and eating healthy, 'clean' food. Many such foods are also considered beneficial for those living with dementia.

FOODS THAT ARE GOOD FOR DEMENTIA AND ALZHEIMER'S DISEASE

A number of foods are said to be good to help prevent Alzheimer's and dementia, and there are some that should be avoided (Hobson 2013). As part of your commitment to sauca, why not make a commitment to include more of these 'clean' foods in your diet from now on?

Foods to include more of in your diet, and why they are good for you

- Green leafy vegetables such as spinach or kale – these contain folate and B12, which can help improve mental functioning and reduce depression.

- Broccoli, cauliflower, avocado and asparagus – these contain folate and carotenoids that help lower amino acid, which is linked to reduced brain functioning.

- Vegetables that are high in vitamin D and iron, such as pumpkin, asparagus, tomatoes, carrots and beetroot, are also good.

- Nuts such as almonds, cashews, walnuts, hazelnuts, peanuts and pecans – these contain a good mix of vitamins, folate and omega oil.

- Berries and cherries contain anthocyanin that protects the brain from further damage caused by free radicals. They also have anti-inflammatory properties and contain antioxidants and lots of vitamin C and E.

- Beans contain folate, iron, magnesium and potassium that can help with general body function and neuron firing. They also contain choline, a B vitamin that boosts acetylcholine, a neurotransmitter that is critical for brain function.

- Whole grains such as quinoa, brown rice and seeds such as sunflower seeds and pumpkin seeds contain zinc, choline and vitamin E.

- Omega 3-containing food, such as olive oil, fish or flaxseeds, is good, or a good omega 3 supplement.

- Spices such as cinnamon, sage, turmeric and cumin are said to help break up brain plaque, and reduce inflammation of the brain.

Eating these foods will also decrease the risks of other illnesses that can make the brain age, such as obesity, heart disease, diabetes and hypertension.

Foods to avoid or reduce

- As well as increasing the above foods, it is advisable to reduce your intake of high-fat, sugary and salty food such as red meat, butter, fried food, salt, pastries and cakes.

- Common foods such as white bread are particularly bad as wheat contains amylopectin A, a type of molecule that is more efficiently converted to blood sugar than just about any other carbohydrate. After eating a slice or two, blood sugar levels increase within two hours, leaving you feeling hungry again. White bread is particularly bad as it is finely ground and stripped of its bran and germ, the elements that contain fibre, vitamins and minerals. Refined grains are low in magnesium, zinc, vitamin E and fibre.

- Excessive sugar in the diet is also particularly bad for those living with dementia. In fact, it has recently been shown to be a potential cause of Alzheimer's disease (Kassaar *et al.* 2017). Furthermore, added sugar contains no essential nutrients that your body needs – it has no protein, essential fats, vitamins or minerals.

- On the subject of what to avoid, smoking and excessive drinking can also contribute to the risk of developing dementia.

Santosha, or contentment. Santosha is about accepting our situation. So, for example if you or a loved one has been diagnosed with dementia, at first you might feel denial and maybe that it is a mistake (see the introduction to Chapter 10). However, with any big life change, once we stop mentally rejecting a situation, we often find inside that we have the capacity to change. Life is filled with a vast mixture of good and bad experiences, and how we deal with adversity and bad times is what really makes us grow as individuals.

To help practise contentment, focus on the good things we have in our lives. So, for example, even if we have had bad news or are having a bad day, we often still have things to be grateful for, such as a comfortable dry bed to sleep in, some beautiful flowers to look at, friends we can talk to etc.

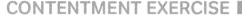

CONTENTMENT EXERCISE

Next time you are having negative thoughts, focus on the good things and write a list of these. This is a powerful practice that can be made part of your daily routine, so either first thing in the morning or just before bed, take five minutes to write down or say five things you are grateful for. If you are working with someone with dementia, ask them to say five things they are grateful for – you could take it in turns saying one thing each. Again, they do not need to be big things, they could be everyday things such as a family member phoning, or a nice meal, or a hug. Many studies have linked feeling more *grateful* with an improved sense of wellbeing, so this seemingly simple exercise can be very powerful.

Tapas, or austerity. The word *tapa* comes from the word to heat, but in particular, the heat needed for birth, or to hatch an egg. It has evolved to mean the 'heat' of spiritual discipline, and can be interpreted as our commitment to transform ourselves and improve our life. A regular yogic practice can take as little as 15–30 minutes a day, so why not make a commitment today to your tapas or yoga practice. This could be as simple as saying that you will spend 15 minutes one day reading this book, and the next day trying one of the simple exercises.

Svadhyaya, or self-study. This is about our spiritual education and learning. We spend so much of our lives looking outwards, and projecting an image of ourselves on to others. Self-study is about countering this by finding out more about our true selves. It can help us release tendencies or habits that are no longer useful. Self-study allows us to observe our reactions, and let go of those reactions we no longer need in life. No matter how old we are, we still have the capacity to learn, to be creative and change. However, in order to do so, we first need to create space for this by letting go of things that no longer serve us, for example, certain habits, ideas etc.

Self-study could take the form of meditation (see 'Journey of awareness' on page 131, Chapter 8), reading an inspiring book and thinking about it, or watching an inspiring and uplifting film, or writing in your notebook.

Isvara prandidhana is about surrendering ourselves to our higher essence or 'god'. Your god does not have to be a 'god' in the traditional sense of the word that refers to a superior being. Your god can be anything you believe in and love, or anything you can focus on – the stars in the sky, the vastness of it all, the sun and its incredible raw energy, the energy that gives us heat in the winter, and the power that helps our fruit and vegetables to grow and gives us flowers in the park. Focus on that incredible biochemistry that makes up a flower – that beautiful flower in your room can be your god, it can be your point of focus. Just dwell on things that are incredibly wondrous and extraordinary in their own way. Focus on any element of nature, let nature be your god, the magnificent mountains in the Alps or the Himalayas, the vast oceans and seas and the amazing life forms contained within. You could focus on your children or grandchildren or the beauty of their smiles. It is not hard; anyone can choose their own god. God is whatever you want him, her or it to be. In Chapter 13, on bhakti yoga, I provide an exercise to help you focus on your 'god'. 'Some other ideas for creating more bhakti in your life' on page 230.

So we have now explored the first two limbs of yoga, the yamas and the niyamas, about our outer and inner lives. A lovely exercise to do with the yamas and niyamas is to choose ten days and each day do one activity related to the yama or niyama. Use your notebook to write down what you did each day, and how you felt afterwards.

3. Asana

An asana is a yoga pose or position of the body. The position should always be steady and comfortable. Asanas were intended to help develop a healthy and peaceful body to enable us to practise the other limbs of yoga, such as breath exercises or meditation. We will explore many asanas throughout this book, but if you would like to try one now, you could practise mountain pose, or tadasana (as described in 'Sun salutation', on page 161, Chapter 9).

4. Pranayama

In my opinion, the next limb of yoga, which is called pranayama, or breathing exercises, is the one where we can get the most noticeable results quickly. *Prana*, in the ancient Indian language Sanskrit, means energy or life force. In Chinese medicine the same energy is referred to as chi, and *ayama* means to direct or control. So pranayama is about increasing, directing and extending our life force. Pranayama can also be viewed as a set of breathing practices that are designed for a specific result. While there are hundreds, if not thousands, of different breathing techniques, in this book we introduce a few of the simplest and most effective methods. Often in modern life we subconsciously hold the breath, and do not make the best use of our breathing capacity.

 A SIMPLE 5-MINUTE BREATHING EXERCISE

Many people who have never learned any breathing techniques have very little breath awareness, and might not even know if they are breathing in or out. This simple breathing exercise will help you develop your breath awareness.

First, take a moment to observe how you feel – for example, your stress levels etc. – and write a note of this in your notebook. Next, take a moment to blow your nose. Now sit or lie down in any comfortable position, making sure you are not wearing a tight belt and your belly is able to move freely. Take your hand on to your belly, and as you breathe in, feel your belly lifting, and as you breathe out, feel your belly moving down. If you are not doing so already, breathe only through your nose. Next, start to count how long your inhale lasts for, and how long you exhale for. Try to count by saying the words like this in your mind: 'Inhale 2, 3, 4, Exhale 2, 3, 4' or 'Breathe in 2, 3, 4, Breathe out 2, 3, 4.' The word 'inhale' or 'breathe in' acts as the first count. The main thing is to be very clear if you are breathing in or out. At first do not try to change the breath; just observe your inhale and exhale for about a minute.

Next, begin to make your exhale longer than your inhale. So if you inhale for 3 counts, exhale for 4–6 counts. It doesn't matter how much longer your exhale is; the key thing is for your breath to be comfortable, and for you not to feel like you are straining the breath, or not getting enough breath. Continue for about another 4 minutes, and then allow your breath to return to normal. Observe how you feel both mentally and physically, and make a note of this.

There are many benefits of breathing together with a friend or a loved one, and when two people are close together, their breath often falls into the same pattern. This is known as 'entrainment of the breath'. Entrainment can also happen when listening to music, or we can become entrained to a faster and more hectic pace of life. As well as speech humans communicate through rhythm, and the breath and heartbeat set our own internal rhythm. At a subtle level breathing together is one of the methods we communicate by. With speech, for instance, conversations tend to naturally follow breathing patterns. However, when speech becomes difficult, other methods of communicating through rhythm can be used, for example, body tapping (see page 220, Chapter 12), breathing together (such as 'Cooling breath' on page 189, Chapter 10) or producing sounds (such as the 'Sea of Oms' exercise on page 222, Chapter 12).

5. Pratyahara

The fifth limb of yoga is pratyahara, or withdrawal of the senses from external objects, and focusing on the internal world. This limb of yoga is very important for people living with dementia, as the external world is likely to become more confusing. In the modern world people can be very external-focused and reactionary. Practising pratyahara can help us all realise that we have a deep internal peaceful place within us that we can retreat to and use as a resource for our happiness and wellbeing.

PRATYAHARA EXERCISE

Close your eyes and take one of your fingertips and press the space between your eyebrows – this is known in yoga as the 'third eye point'. Then, with your eyes still closed, see if you can keep all your focus and attention on this point. See if you can allow thoughts and sounds to cease, and just focus on this point.

6. Dharana

The sixth limb of yoga is dharana, or one-pointed focus. This stage develops the previous step as the mind becomes very focused on one thing. This could be, for example, the sound of the word 'om', an image of our personal 'god' or anything you would like to focus on. Once I was in a group with a meditation teacher and a number of other pupils. One student, Anil, a wealthy businessman from Sydney, Australia, told the teacher that he was having real problems remaining focused on any one thing, as he would always be distracted by thoughts of his businesses and money! The teacher then told him that he should make money the focus of his meditation and in particular, a bar of gold bullion. The next week we met again in the meditation group, and the teacher asked him how his practice was going. He said it was much better and he was able to keep the image of the gold bullion in his mind a lot longer than any other image, and his focus and business dealings had improved. This example shows that we do not have to use an image of a 'person' as a point of focus; we can use anything important to us that has meaning.

   DHARANA EXERCISE

Choose something or someone important to you to focus on. If you have a physical image, you could gaze at this first, and then close your eyes. Try to form a mental image of them or it in your mind. See if you can really focus your attention on all aspects of the being or thing. Try to keep this image in your mind for as long as possible. If the image fades, re-open your eyes to look at the picture of the object, if you are using one, again.

If you are not sure what to focus on, you could use this image of the Sri Yantra. The Sri Yantra is a symbol that is many thousands of years old. A yantra is a form of sacred geometry, and is said to bring many benefits, including healing benefits, to those who meditate on it. It has a mathematically precise design that is based on the pi ratio, which relates to the golden proportion.

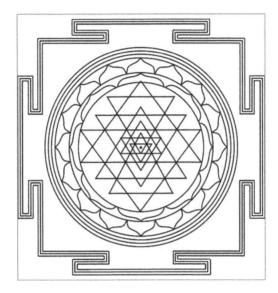

For people living with the later stages of dementia, a good way of engaging with the Sri Yantra is to print out a black and white copy of the image and colour it in as a group activity. Now at first blush you might think that colouring is something that might be seen as patronising for those living with dementia, but what you might not know is that there has been a huge growth in sacred geometry colouring books for adults, and these are said to be highly relaxing and help with meditation practices. The creation of sacred images is used all over the world, from Tibetan monks creating intricate mandalas with sand to Native Americans creating medicine wheels. Mandalas, yantras and colouring sacred geometry images can help bring harmony, unity and healing.

7. Dhyana

The seventh limb of yoga is known as dhyana. Dhyana means contemplation, reflection and profound, abstract meditation. Performing dhyana is about meditating on a point of focus, with the intention of knowing the truth about it. It is when our previous practices of focus become more of a state of flow, which is when we are fully absorbed in an activity. According to the Yoga Sutra, the purpose of meditation is about interrupting the fluctuations of normal mental activity such as sensory knowledge, memory and imagination. It is said that of these, memory is the hardest sense to make quiet, as whenever we sit still, memories will pop up and surface, along with thoughts and things from our 'to do' list. However, the mind is like another muscle in the body, and it has great capacity to adapt and change.

Like any other limb in yoga, meditation is a systematic process in itself, which takes practice to learn. It is like taming a puppy that would much rather run around than sit still. You will need to train your mind to come back to you and the present moment when you tell it to, and to sit still, even if for just a few seconds at a time. Guided relaxations are often a great way to start meditation. The yoga nidra exercise outlined on page 234, Chapter 14, is a wonderful guided meditation/relaxation, and can be a great way of practising focus and concentration with those living with the later stages of dementia.

8. Samadhi

This is the eighth limb of yoga, sometimes known as bliss or nirvana, a state of meditative consciousness. It is a meditative absorption or trance, which is reached through practising the above stages. Sometimes it can be achieved spontaneously. Yogic thought believes that a person is more than just the collection of their mental and physical faculties, and that underneath there is a presence (sometimes called a soul). Samadhi is when we uncover the perfect and shining nature of the soul, and merge with the universal soul. In this state the idea of the individual self dissolves.

As well as the eight limbs of yoga there are a number of other important elements of yoga philosophy. This book touches on these briefly now to provide the background about why we do certain practices, and the philosophical ideas about how they work.

KOSHAS, THE ENERGY SHEATHS OF THE BODY

Yogis believe that the body has a number of layers ranging from the outer 'gross' layers to the inner more subtle and fine layers. These layers or sheaths fit inside the actual space of the body and can be accessed by our deeper layers of consciousness. The *annamaya kosha* is the gross physical body, made up of blood and muscles. We can help protect and strengthen it by doing asanas and other physical exercises. The *pranamaya kosha* is the energy sheath made up of prana or chi. We can protect and strengthen this through breathing exercises. The *manomaya kosha* is made up of the mind stuff or conscious thoughts. We can strengthen and protect this through meditation. The *vijnanamaya kosha* is known as the wisdom sheath. We can protect and strengthen this by observing the yamas and niyamas. The last sheath is the *anandamaya kosha*, and this is the bliss sheath. In yoga philosophy it is considered that our true nature is one of bliss, and in life this is often hidden by the ego and our mental preoccupations. We can practise accessing the bliss body by focusing on selfless activities and practising bhakti yoga (see Chapter 13).

TAMAS, RAJA AND SATTVA, BALANCING THE ELEMENTS

It is believed in yogic thinking that we all have within us three main types of energy called gunas: tamas, rajas and sattva. *Tamas* is the energy of inertia; it is when we feel lazy and lack energy. *Rajas* is a dynamic frantic energy and change. *Sattva* is a balanced energy and brings us to a state of harmony and peace. It is the sattvic energy that those on the yogic path aim for. Many of the exercises in this book aim to help readers balance their energies, for example, tree pose (vriksasana) on page 67, Chapter 4.

THE NADIS OR ENERGY CHANNELS

Ancient yogis, both in India and Tibet, believe that the body contains thousands of energy channels known as nadis. There are different numbers of energy channels quoted, but the most often is 72,000. These correspond to both physical channels such as the veins and nerves, and also the unseen 'cosmic' channels that carry energy known as prana, thoughts and other subtle sensations. Of these nadis three are the most important, and these are known as ida, pingali and sushuama. *Ida* is related to the moon and feminine qualities, and in this respect it is related to tamas above; it is also related to right-brain activities such as creativity and the arts. *Pingali* relates to the sun and masculine qualities related to logic and sciences. *Sushuama* is generally associated with the brain and spinal column, and it is said that when our energy flows freely in the sushuama we are in a balanced and calm state. Again, the alternate nostril breathing (nadi shodhana) exercises on page 208, Chapter 11, help to balance the nadis.

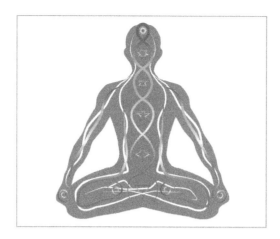

Along the spine it is believed that there are also seven major energy centres known as the chakras. These are said to be spinning balls of energy, but they also largely correspond to the major nerve clusters that come out of the spine. These various clusters of nerves play a very important role in transmitting information from the brain to the various essential organs contained in the torso. The following diagram shows how the major clusters of organs correspond to the chakras.

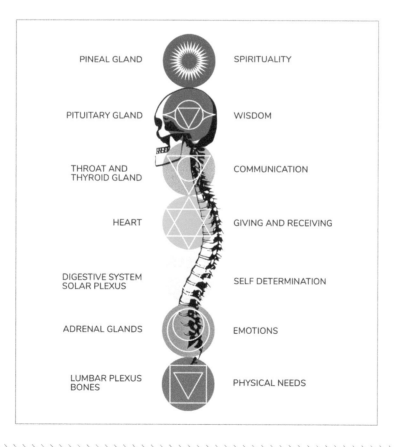

Whilst it is not necessary to know that much about chakras to do the exercises in this book, it is useful to know that these energy centres can become blocked. This might manifest in us feeling a bit out of balance or with more specific problems such as difficulties communicating, or shutting off our emotions. The exercises in this book, in particular, the alternate nostril breathing (nadi shodhana) exercise in Chapter 11, page 208 and sun salutation (surya namaskar) in Chapter 9, page 161, will help you connect and realign your essential energy centres.

CONCLUSION

This chapter has provided a brief introduction to some of the key aspects of yoga philosophy. Whilst it is not necessary to know anything about yoga philosophy to practise yoga, I find that having some knowledge about the reasons we do certain things and the thoughts behind them make them more meaningful for all of those involved in the activities and practices.

CHAPTER 4

YOGA BASICS AND SIMPLE EVERYDAY POSES

In previous chapters we have explored the different types of yoga and some key aspects of yoga philosophy. We now look at how we can put these basic principles of yoga into practice by exploring some simple breathing exercises, asanas and restful and restorative poses, which will help you to understand more about what yoga is.

Yoga is an experiential practice, meaning that we can read all we like in books about the benefits of yoga, but it is only when we experience them ourselves that we can really understand the practice of yoga. In this chapter I provide a range of practices that are suitable for those living with dementia, their carers and relatives. While these practices together form a 'foundations of yoga' sequence, those you are working with could also enjoy one or two of these simple everyday poses as part of a shorter practice. These exercises can be done at any time.

SIMPLE BREATHING EXERCISES

    ### THREE-PART BREATH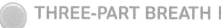

Three-part breath, also sometimes known as full yogic breath, is one of the simplest yet most effective breathing exercises. We have seen that when we are tense our breath tends to be fast, shallow and ragged. When we are relaxed we breathe slowly and deeply. Many people do not realise the benefits of good breathing. In fact, when I tell people that I teach breathing exercises, I often get the response, 'What do you mean, you teach breathing techniques – we all know how to breathe, otherwise we'd be dead!' However, for many people, the breath is tight,

restricted and shallow, a term known as 'frozen breathing'. In these cases a person might hold the outer shell and muscles of their body tightly, which restricts the inner movements of the body (Farhi 1996).

Some people have little awareness of their breath and might find it difficult to distinguish if they are breathing in or out. Three-part breath helps everyone to 'make friends' with their breath by getting to know it a bit better. It might sound corny, but in my experience, the breath is one of our greatest teachers – it is with us from the moment we are born to the moment we die. It is a constant wave or cycle within us, and when we learn to connect with it, it can help us. It is free, readily available and can bring so many wonderful benefits. If you are cynical or have doubts about breathing practices, do give breath work a try as it is an essential part of yoga – I think you will be pleasantly surprised by its effects.

Three-part breath can be done lying down or sitting up straight. As in corpse pose (shavasana) (see page 72, later in this chapter), make sure your spine is straight and your body is symmetrical by ensuring your arms and legs are placed an even distance from the torso and your head is in line with your spine.

Place your hands right down on your lower belly, so that your little fingers touch the top of the hips. Spread the fingers wide and have the tips of the middle finger lightly touching. As you breathe in and out through your nose, see if you can direct the breath into your belly. As you breathe deeper into your belly, see if you can feel the tips of the middle fingers move apart – this might only be by about 5 millimetres or a centimetre. This doesn't matter – the key thing is that the breath is going into the belly and the belly is relaxed.

When we are truly relaxed we naturally breathe deep into our belly; however, many people, due to the pressure of society to have a flat belly, or clothes that are perhaps too tight, never really relax their belly, which leads to poor breathing habits. So as you relax, try to tap into the feeling of the belly gently moving up and down.

After spending 2 to 3 minutes like this, move your hands to either side of your ribs. Spread your fingers and press your hands gently into the side of the ribs so you can feel them moving as you breathe in and out. Be aware of the breath moving the ribs, and see if you can feel the way the breath not only lifts the ribs, but also moves them out to the side and presses the ribs into the back of the floor. Try to imagine that the breath is filling up the lungs like a balloon. Stay like this for 2 to 3 minutes.

Next, bring your hands up to your collarbones, spread the fingers wide so the little fingers almost touch the sternum (breastbone) and the thumbs the inside edge of the shoulders, and focus on the breath moving in the upper chest. Feel how the breastbone lifts as you inhale, and as you exhale allow the shoulders to move out and down. Again, stay like this for 2 to 3 minutes.

Next, bring your right hand down to the belly and leave the left hand where it is. Feel the breath first arising in the belly, next the ribs, and then into the upper hand. Then feel the breath leave the upper chest, mid-chest and then the belly.

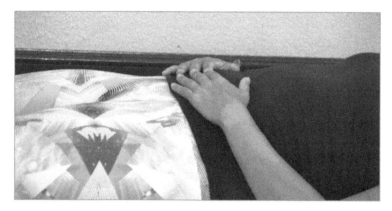

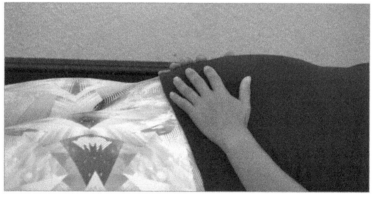

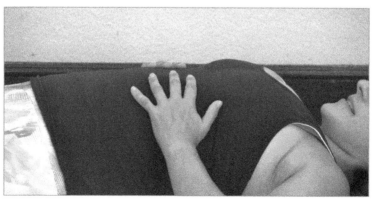

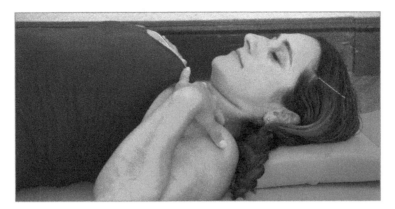

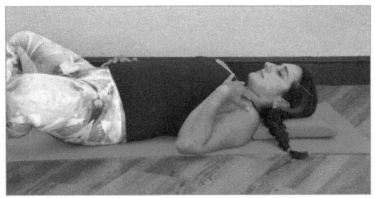

It can be helpful to imagine that the torso is an empty vessel and we are drinking in the breath through a straw, filling the torso from bottom to top. On the out-breath you could imagine the breath is like a gas and it evaporates from the lungs from the top to the bottom. Spend 5 minutes just focusing on this full, deep, yogic breath. If you find your mind wandering, you could introduce an even breath count, that is, counting 4–6 as you inhale and the same number on the exhale. Remember never to strain or force the breath.

After finishing the three-part breath, return to a natural breath for a minute or so, and take some time to tune in with yourself and note how you feel. If you are working with a person or a group, encourage them to come out of this practice gently, to open their eyes and stretch. Try to ensure during the practice that the light in the room is soft, so when you or they open their eyes the contrast is not too great as this can be particularly disorientating for those living with dementia.

UJJAYI BREATH

Ujjayi breath is sometimes known as the victorious breath or the ocean breath. It can be practised as a stand-alone breathing exercise or combined with movements in traditional yoga. It helps to reduce blood pressure and can bring more oxygen to the lungs. As with any pranayama (breathing) technique, ujjayi should never be strained, and if you feel like you are not getting enough air, always just return to a natural breath. Ujjayi breath is a lovely breath to do when we are feeling stressed or anxious, and we can use it as a self-medicine, or with someone we are working with.

The benefits of full yogic breath include the fact that it engages the three main parts of the lungs and can help to correct poor breathing patterns. It also helps to release stress and activates the rest and restore mode of the body.

To start, sit in a comfortable position with a straight back. Take a deep breath in, and then breathe out through your mouth, like you are cleaning a pair of glasses, misting a mirror or warming your hands on a cold day, making a gentle 'haaaa' sound. You can hold your hand up to your mouth so you can feel the breath. Try this a few times and feel the sensation that this type of breath makes in the throat. You should feel a little vibration and hear a sound like a distant wave, hence the name 'ocean breath'.

Try breathing out a few times with your mouth open and making the gentle 'haaaa' sound. Next time you breathe out through your mouth, close your lips halfway through the exhale breath. Try to continue feeling the vibration and hear the sound with your mouth closed. Next, see if you can keep making this sound as you breathe in as well as when you breathe out, so that you have a constant sound like a wave in your throat.

Once you have got the idea, practise ujjayi breath for 2 to 5 minutes using one of the mudras below. Try alternating between practising it very quietly and practising it loudly. Eventually find a way to practise it gently, so that it sounds like a distant wave. Take a moment to see the effects of the breath on your mood and mental chatter.

MUDRAS AND BALANCING EXERCISES

A mudra is a hand or body gesture that is designed to change the subtle energetic balance of our bodies. Mudras can be part of our asana practice, but can also be used in meditation practices. Through using the hands, mudras stimulate meridian and reflexology points in the hands. They also provide a place where we can focus our attention. I now introduce you to two very useful mudras.

GYAN MUDRA

One of the most popular mudras is gyan mudra, which is also known as the mudra of knowledge. It is said to help ease tension and depression and is related to expansion and knowledge. It is very calming and helps to open us to new experiences. This mudra can be used in any meditation or guided relaxations.

To perform this mudra, sit in a comfortable position. Rest your hands on your knees, and put the tips of the first finger and thumb together. If you are feeling more energetic, you can rest the hands with your palm down on your knees, or if you are tired, you can rest with the palms facing up.

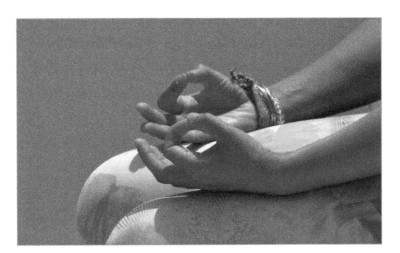

DHYANI MUDRA

Another simple and common mudra is dhyani mudra, the mudra of receiving, which I have often found useful when studying or learning. You could use this mudra as a learning tool when you read something in this book that you'd like to take in or remember. This is also commonly used in meditation – our hands form an empty bowl shape, which signifies openness and acceptance of what we are going to receive. This can be used when listening or reading, or simply to relax the hands.

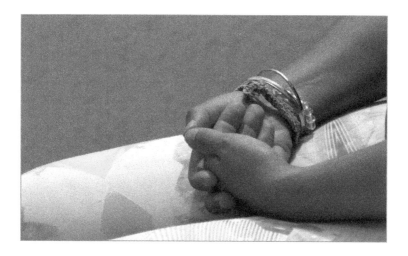

Place your hands in your lap with your palms facing up. Next, place your left hand on top of your right hand and have the tips of your thumbs lightly touching. Rest the hands softly down in your lap.

You can practise gyan or dhyani mudra at the same time as practising ujjayi breath.

TREE POSE, VRIKSASANA

We can all sometimes feel like a tree being buffeted by a storm, especially when we are going through a difficult period in our lives. This simple tree pose is a balancing pose. Balancing poses are great for bringing our awareness out of our heads and into our bodies. They also help to improve focus and concentration and help us 'find our feet' after receiving difficult news. After my dad died whilst I was in my final year of university, I found that balances were one of the few things that really took my mind away from the pain and grief.

When I introduce balances to groups, I will often get people saying to me, 'Oh I'm rubbish at balances.' But what people do not realise is that if we can walk, we can balance, because the act of walking requires us to be constantly on one leg or the other. And if you feel balancing is difficult, then you really should be practising this exercise to help improve it.

Tree pose can be practised regularly, and it can be part of a general yoga practice; for example, it can be combined with the sun salutations (see page 161, Chapter 9), or as a stand-alone exercise.

The benefits of balance poses include improved focus and concentration, building up the muscles in the legs and feet, improved core strength and improved awareness of our position in space. As balances are great for increasing focus and bodily awareness, this will benefit those living with the early stages of dementia.

Stand tall in mountain pose, or tadasana (page 161), with your feet firmly placed under the hips – bare feet is best for this exercise. If you feel like your balance is not good, use a wall or the back of a chair to support you, in which case, stand side on to it. Wiggle and spread your toes and place them back down on the floor or mat. Next, close your eyes and take your weight gradually forwards and backwards, and from side to side. Try to notice the balance of the body shifting and how different parts of the body work when you are leaning forwards or backwards. Continue until you feel that you are standing right over the centre of your feet – if you had a plumb line it would go straight down from the crown of your head to the middle of your feet.

Next, imagine you are growing roots under both your feet, like a very tall tree – visualise many roots going deep and wide. Find a point about 1–1.5 metres in front of you on the floor to focus on – it should be something that is not moving.

Press down into your left foot, lift your right foot and place the sole of the right foot on to your left ankle. If you are using a wall or chair, use your left hand to gently support you. Try to feel the way the body makes constant adjustments in order to balance. If you feel confident, try closing your eyes for a moment to feel these micro-adjustments more. Try not to be scared or stiffen when you feel these little movements; instead, breathe slowly and deeply, feel into your feet and imaginary roots, and imagine you are a tree swaying in a gentle breeze.

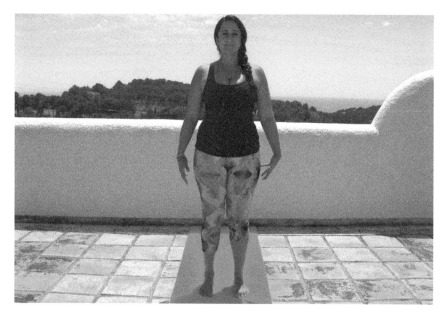

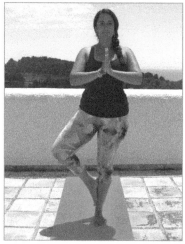

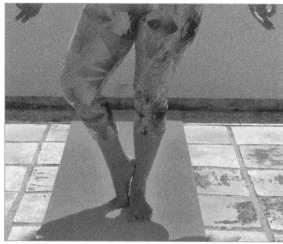

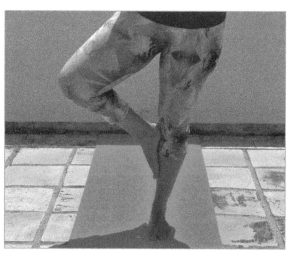

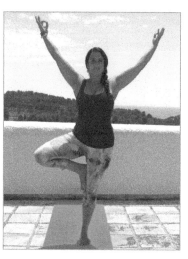

If you would like to you can lift your right foot higher up the leg to your shin or thigh (but never rest the foot on the knee as this can cause knee pain). Your knee should be pointing out to the right.

If you are not supporting yourself with a chair or wall, bring your hands to the heart with the palms together at the heat centre in a prayer pose (angali mudra, the mudra of greeting) and take a few breaths. If you feel stable, bring this prayer pose above your head, or extend both arms up to the sky and feel like they are branches lifting to the sun.

When you have finished practising on the right side, take your leg and arms down. Give your legs and ankles a shake to release any tension. Then, when you are ready, repeat the exercise on the left-hand side. Try to notice if one side is easier than the other.

After you have finished both sides, either rest in mountain pose (tadasana) or lie down in corpse pose (shavasana, page 76) and then make a note of how you feel.

NATURAL EASY STRETCHES

PUSHING AWAY THE CLOUDS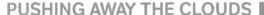

Pushing away the clouds is a fantastic pose that can be done at any time. It is great for the arms, hands and shoulders, but is also fantastic if we feel like everything is getting on top of us and we are lacking personal space. It helps us locate our body in space, which is often one of the things that goes when we are living with dementia.

Pushing away the clouds can be done from a sitting or standing position. First, start with the palms together at the heart centre, in angali mudra, the mudra of greeting (prayer pose; see page 67). Press the thumbs gently into the sternum. Take a moment to notice how you are feeling.

Next, imagine you are pushing something away – start to push out in front of you with your palms facing forwards. Then exhale and push out to the sides. You can push all around with the hands together or out in separate directions. See if you can push all the way around you, including pushing away behind you.

Each time you push, use some resistance in your arms to feel like you are pushing away soft spongy clouds. Creating this resistance helps work the arms, chest and shoulder muscles more.

When you have finished pushing away your imaginary clouds, stand in the centre of your space with your hands back in prayer pose. Close your eyes and see if you can feel the space you have created around you.

NATURAL MORNING STRETCHES

When I watch children and animals move, I am often inspired by the way that they seem to incorporate stretching into their everyday routines. When a cat or dog wakes up it will often perform yoga-like stretches; toddlers and young children also seem to delight in the movements and possibilities of their bodies. However, as we age, we often seem to forget the natural joy of moving. Natural varied movements and stretches help to stretch our interconnective tissue. Some research (Headly 2009) refers to this interconnective tissue as 'fuzz' that builds up overnight and needs to be stretched and massaged by movement for its optimal functionality. This makes up lines along the body that can be stretched and strengthened by various yoga poses. Stretches help lengthen the side of the body.

Here is an exercise to stretch our interconnective tissue. It is a more restorative pose and is performed either lying down or on a chair.

In the lying down (or supine) position, begin by lying on your back, on a yoga mat or blanket. You can also do this position in bed. Next, keeping your shoulders and hips on the floor, stretch your arms up over your head so they ideally touch the floor behind you; you can bend your elbows.

Take hold of your left wrist with your right hand. Then move your arms and feet over to the right, being careful to keep your hips and shoulders on the floor. You can take little steps with your ankles to shuffle your feet along.

For an intensive stretch in the side of your leg, cross your left ankle over your right ankle. You should feel a nice stretch in the right side of your body. Stay here for a few breaths. Next, shuffle your feet back to the centre and move your arms back to the centre. Take your arms down by your sides and rest for a while.

See if you can notice any difference in the feeling in the right side of your body.

Repeat the exercise on the left side. Remember to rest at the end in a symmetrical position (see page 62).

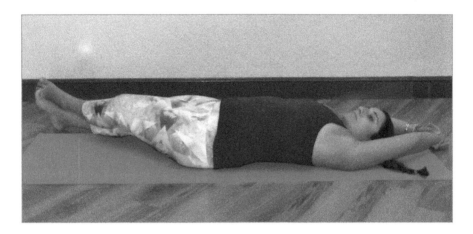

If you would like to add another level to this exercise, you can perform it for 3 to 5 minutes on each side while practising three-part breath at the same time (see page 61).

In the next exercise we explore moving our spine and stretching our back.

   ## CAT AND COW

As well as stretching the spine, cat and cow also mobilises and stretches the hips and abdomen. Moving with the breath helps to increase our coordination. Cat and cow also massages our internal organs including our belly, kidneys and adrenal glands. It can be done from a number of starting positions, but is most often taught from an all-fours position.

First, come on to your hands and knees with your hands under your shoulders, arms straight and knees under your hips. Next, inhale and lift your head and tailbone up to the ceiling, at the same time dropping your belly towards the floor – your body will be curving towards the floor. As you then exhale, suck your belly in and lift it towards the ceiling, at the same time dropping your head and tailbone and looking towards your belly – your back will be arching up towards the ceiling. Repeat this movement four to ten times, moving with the breath and really feeling into the body on each inhale and exhale.

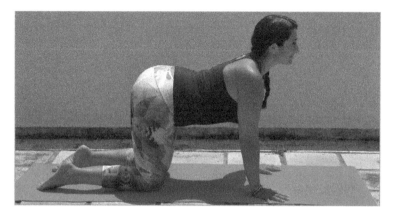

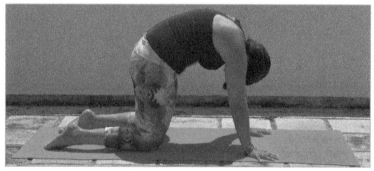

This pose can also be done from sitting or standing – inhale, arch your head and shoulders back, at the same time pushing your waist forwards so you stretch your spine, then exhale, pull your belly in and curve your spine.

RESTORATIVE POSES

Restorative poses are yoga positions that are held longer than normal poses. They often work with gravity and deep meditative breathing, to slowly release and unwind. Restorative yoga helps you to turn inward, focus on the breath and release tension.

 LEGS UP THE WALL, VIPARITA KARANI

I consider legs up the wall one of the best restorative poses. It is perfect for those living with the early stages of dementia, and is also great for carers and family members, or those who spend a lot of time on their feet.

An easier version can also be done from lying down in a bed, so people in later-stage dementia, or those who cannot get into the full position, can also benefit. It is most effective when it is combined with mindful breathing, such as three-part breath or simple breath awareness (see page 61).

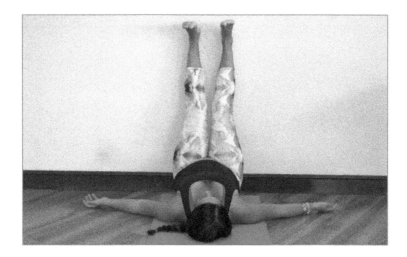

When we are on our feet a lot, our body, and in particular, our hearts and the veins in our legs, have to work quite hard to pump blood all the way back up to our hearts. When our legs are higher than our heart, gravity can help return the blood and lymphatic fluid back to the heart. This can help improve swelling, improve circulation and the condition of varicose veins. Having the legs elevated has a number of other benefits including reducing blood pressure, and it is said to help relieve depression. It can also help sufferers of peripheral arterial disease – when narrowed arteries reduce blood supply to the limbs. And it can help reduce atherosclerosis, the hardening and narrowing of the arteries. It can be used as a 'rescue remedy' for fatigue and exhaustion, and can help to turn on the rest and restore mode of the nervous system. It should, however, be avoided if you have glaucoma or high blood pressure, or if you have serious neck or spine issues.

To do the full version of legs up the wall, take your yoga mat and place it side on to a wall. If you do not have a yoga mat you can just use a section of carpeted floor or a rug, but be careful not to lie on a cold floor, or on a potentially slippery surface. You can also take a towel or a blanket and fold it a few times so that it is approximately

12 inches or 30 centimetres long, or at least the width of your body. Leave this to the side for now.

Next, sit on the floor, with your hip next to the wall. Then lie down, swinging your legs and feet up the wall. Your back and head should be on the floor. Once you have swung your legs up the wall you might find that your bottom has moved away from the wall. Use your elbows and shuffle your sit bones towards the wall, taking your legs as far up the wall as comfortable, and moving as close to the wall as possible. If you like, push the soles of your feet into the wall and lift your bottom up. Take your folded-up blanket and place it under your hips. You can use pillows or folded-up blankets to lift the hips up and support the hips and buttocks.

If you are unable to get up and down from the floor easily, this position can be done from lying in bed. Either do this yourself, or have someone to help you lift your legs about 8–12 inches above your heart.

Whatever position you are in, set a timer for 10–20 minutes and stay in this position, focusing on a breathing or meditation exercise, such as journey of awareness (see Chapter 8, page 131) or three-part breath (see page 61).

When it is time to come out of the pose, if your legs are up the wall, bend your knees and gently shuffle your bottom away from the wall. Then hug your knees to your chest and roll over to one side, supporting your head with your hands in a foetal position. Rest here for a few minutes and then, when you are ready, come up to sitting.

RECLINED BOUND ANGLE POSE, SUPTA BADDHA KONASANA, WITH SELF-RECHARGE HAND POSITION

Another fantastic restorative pose to do is reclined bound angle pose, or supta baddha konasana. Again, this can be done from lying down or in a bed. This pose helps to open the front of the chest, creating more room to breathe. It can also benefit the heart and improve general circulation. It is also said to be good for stress and depression.

First, elevate the top half of your body by lying on some pillows or folded blankets. Ideally your chin should be higher than your hips and it should be tucked in slightly so that the front of the throat is not extended. Next, take the soles of your feet together and allow your knees to drop out to the side. You can support the knees with a pillow or cushion under each. Try to make sure that each knee is even. Take one hand to your belly and the other to your heart; this is known as self-recharge hand position. In this position you can focus on the flow of breath from the belly to the heart area. If you want to deepen this practice, you can also perform three-part breath (see page 61) for 5 or so minutes while in the pose. Stay in this pose for 5–10 minutes.

To come out of the pose use your hands to help close your thighs or stretch out one leg at a time. Roll over to one side and rest here for a few minutes. Next, use your hands to walk yourself up to sitting.

 ## CORPSE POSE, SHAVASANA

One of the key yoga poses is corpse pose, or shavasana. This is a great resting pose, and you can perform it any time throughout this book. I recommend giving corpse pose a try any time while you are reading the next few chapters, as it is a great way of resting and taking in information. It can be done at the start or end of any yoga practice, or between doing the poses, and is a great way of resting and letting the body's energy rebalance.

Corpses have a special significance in yoga. Shiva, the mythological founder of yoga, was heartbroken when his first wife Sati died. When in mourning he was said to spend many months in the cremation grounds by the banks of the river Ganges, meditating on death.

Practising corpse pose is one of the ways we can prepare our body and mind for death and dying. It is a process of undoing, rather than doing. In one of the classical ancient Indian epic stories, The Mahabharata, a central character, King Yudhishthira, was asked what was the most amazing thing in life. He replied that it was 'That a man, while seeing others die around him, behaves as if he will never die'. Many ancient societies believe that a healthy relationship with dying helps us to live a more meaningful and fulfilled life. Stephen Jenkinson, in his book Die Wise (Jenkinson 2015), talks about the importance of recognising both our own mortality and that of those we care for. Having a healthy relationship with death includes not shying away from talking about dying, making plans with our relatives, and making memories.

To do this pose correctly, lie flat on your back on a comfortable surface (either on a mat or blanket), have your feet wider than your hips, and allow your toes to turn out and your feet to relax completely. Have your arms at about a 45-degree angle from your body or roughly halfway between your hips and your shoulders, with palms turned up. Roll your shoulder blades down your back to make space for your neck.

Lift your head to look down your body and check that your body is symmetrical. Relax your neck by turning your head from side to side, and use a pillow under your head if you need to. If you wear glasses, take them off, putting them carefully to the side. Stretch out your hands and then squeeze them into fists. Now relax them. Stretch your face and then again, relax it. Allow yourself to relax into the blanket or mat. With each exhale imagine you are sinking deeper into the floor – you could almost imagine that your body is melting. With each inhale imagine you are bringing in new energy and healing to the body.

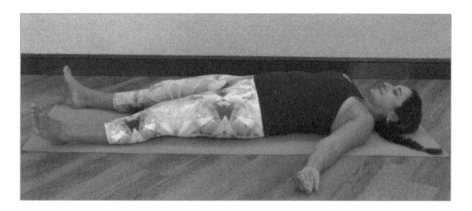

CONCLUSION

In this chapter we have explored a sequence of foundational/simple everyday yoga exercises that combine some simple breathing, balancing exercises and stretches. You might like to try either the whole sequence or a few of the poses by yourself, or with someone you care for. These will help prepare you and your body for later practices in this book. Now you have had an introduction to some of the practical poses, we go on to explore more about why yoga is so beneficial, and for older people in particular.

CHAPTER 5

WHY YOGA IS BENEFICIAL FOR OLDER PEOPLE

When we grow older our bodies and minds change in various ways. In this chapter we look at what happens to older bodies. We explore some of the leading evidence, and examples as to how yoga can help with various facets of ageing. We also briefly touch on how the exercises and sequences contained within this book can help counter the effects of ageing. Chapter 6 then looks at yoga and dementia in more depth.

How we view ageing can be based on a number of facets, for example:

- chronological age – the number of years since birth

- biological age – based on the functional capacity of organs

- psychological age – the adaptive capacity compared to those of the same chronological age

- social age – expected roles in society based on ageing.

(Telles 2016)

All of these factors have a huge impact on how old we feel, or how we perceive the age of others. It is also interesting that only our chronological age is absolute, and not impacted by social or lifestyle choices. The other three factors, biological, psychological and social, are very dependent on the lifestyle choices we make. In fact, so-called 'lifestyle diseases', in particular, those caused by smoking, diet, lack of physical activity, loneliness and stress, are some of the biggest growing causes of morbidity and poor health in the western world. Lifestyle choices are also being increasingly shown to be a contributing factor in diseases such as type 2 diabetes, hypertension, cardiovascular disease and several types of cancer (Golubic 2013).

Illness and disease can play a huge factor in how old we feel, and our ability to maintain strength and positive habits. As people live longer, and worldwide mortality declines, there has been an increase in people living with two or more types of illness or disease. In medical terminology this is known as 'co-morbidities', meaning two illnesses co-existing, and 'multi-morbidities' for more than two illnesses, for example, someone who might have diabetes, high blood pressure and heart disease.

In developed nations, about one in four adults has at least two chronic conditions, and more than half of older adults have three or more chronic conditions (Whitson *et al.* 2016). These other diseases and illnesses combine to limit lifestyle choices, and once a person has one illness or disease, they are often more susceptible and less able to recover from subsequent illnesses.

Many of these diseases are preventable, and health services around the world are looking at how we can reduce the incidence of multiple diseases and premature deaths, and how we can live well for longer. For example, heart disease, cancer and stroke risk are some of the biggest causes of premature mortality in the US (Centers for Disease Control and Prevention Newsroom 2014), and are negatively affected by lack of physical activity. This is why yoga can be so critical to helping us all live well for longer. As I show in this book it is a practice that can be done by anyone, inside or outside, with little or no equipment.

This gives cause for hope, because, as so many illnesses and diseases are impacted by lifestyle choices, there is much we can do to improve our lives and control our own health as we age. In the west, many people increasingly rely on the medical profession to 'fix them'. The increased prevalence of lifestyle diseases, and knowledge about the role of stress in disease, should act as a wake-up call for all of us to take more responsibility for our own health. Yoga is a holistic practice – meaning that it does not separate out parts of the body, or divide the mental and the physical. As a result it works on the whole body and mind, and is therefore extremely beneficial for those with multiple illnesses.

Personal responsibility, action and enquiry are some of the key tenets of yogic philosophy. Yoga can help address some of the lifestyle diseases outlined above through ensuring our bodies and minds are well. However, much 'modern' yoga has put an emphasis on difficult physical positions. In fact, the real goal of the yoga asanas (positions) is to keep our bodies healthy to enable us to sit comfortably in meditative positions.

The practices outlined in this book draw from traditional yoga, but are adapted to suit older people and those living with dementia. Regardless of our age or physical condition, the exercises in this book enable us to take responsibility for our own health and for that of our loved ones and the people we care for, and it is never too late to start. They are gentle and many are suitable for people with illnesses and pre-existing conditions. However, as always, please consult your doctor if you have any pre-existing conditions.

HOW WE AGE PHYSICALLY, AND WHAT HAPPENS TO OUR BODY

Dementia mainly affects the over-65s, and often people living with dementia might have other age-related conditions or diseases. Therefore, in order to look at how yoga can help with dementia, we first need to ask what happens to our bodies, muscles and cells in general as we get older. What happens to our brains? What about our bones? Are these changes inevitable? Or can yoga help keep our bodies and brains healthy? We first take a general look at some of the key things that we might start noticing as we get older, and this will help us understand how yoga and meditation practices can help.

Decline in energy levels and weakness

One of the first signs of ageing might be a feeling of losing strength. Whilst there are some physical reasons for this, including a decreased muscle to fat ratio, becoming weaker is not an inevitable part of ageing. Providing a person remains fit and active, ageing alone reduces muscle mass and strength by no more than about 10 to 15 per cent during an adult's lifetime. We all know that when the body is inactive, muscle mass quickly declines, and this gets worse as we get older. For example, to make up for the muscle mass lost during each day of strict bed rest, older people may need to exercise for up to two weeks after.

Much decline in muscle mass and energy can be related to sedentary lifestyles. In the developed world, people are spending more and more time in environments that limit physical activity and require prolonged sitting, for example, at work, home, in a car, playing computer games, etc. Furthermore, work environments such as offices, schools, homes and public spaces have been re-engineered in ways that minimise human movement and muscular activity. For example, the increasing prevalence of household electronic goods, the use of escalators and lifts and the ease of transport options means that people do not have to do so much physical work in the house, walking generally, or walking up stairs.

Yoga helps to mimic natural movements, and takes the spine and body through a whole range of movements, thereby providing the body with a complete range of activity. Yoga often combines both aerobic, strength-building exercises and stretches, thereby helping to counter the effects of a sedentary lifestyle.

In some cases, lower energy levels and weight loss can result in frailty, which is a common syndrome in older people. There are a number of risk factors that contribute to frailty including disease, physiologic impairments or increased stress hormones. Another thing that often happens with ageing is a loss of flexibility, including joint disorders such as arthritis. This can lead to moving becoming painful and a subsequent reduction in movement and further stiffening of joints. Yoga helps to increase flexibility, decreases stress hormones and can help reduce inflammation associated with arthritis. While historically advice to those with arthritis was to limit movement, more up-to-date recommendations are to move the body where possible to reduce further decline in the possibility and range of movements.

When we age, we often lose bone density, which can result in osteoporosis. This is a thinning of the bones and it happens when bone loss outpaces the growth of new bones. Bones become porous, brittle and prone to fracture. This can be a particular problem for older people as they become more susceptible to injuries, and when they are injured, they take longer to heal. This often results in a loss of confidence in movement, leading to further decline. Again, yoga can help; in particular, it can provide gentle weight-bearing exercises to help keep bones healthy.

Frailty, osteoporosis and depression (see below) can also result in chronic pain, including types of pain such as lower back, neck or shoulder pain that may be the result of poor posture or repetitive strain injury (RSI). Yoga helps to improve posture. A real example of this was the case of Anna Pesce who started yoga when she was 85. Anna had quite poor posture and really bad scoliosis (curvature of her spine), a herniated disc and osteoporosis. After working with a specialised yoga teacher, Rachel Jesien, for nine months, she managed to completely transform her posture.

A balanced yoga practice, by providing a range of movements, also helps to avoid issues such as RSI. And people have learned to associate less with their pain through various meditation techniques, which can often lessen its impact.

Many people might find themselves putting on weight as they get older. Middle-aged spread or abdominal obesity is strongly linked to impaired glucose tolerance and insulin sensitivity. Impaired glucose tolerance comes with an increased risk of cardiovascular disease and likelihood of developing diabetes. A physical yoga practice that gets people moving and increases people's heart rates can help to reduce weight gain. Yoga is also often combined with mindfulness, which involves watching our reactions and examining our habits. Through this we can practise a more balanced approach to eating.

Many older people tend to find that they sleep less and their sleep quality becomes poorer. Often people might find themselves going to bed earlier and getting up earlier. Insomnia and disrupted sleep can lead to feeling more tired in the daytime. Untreated sleep apnoea puts a person at risk for cardiovascular disease, headaches, memory loss and depression. Yoga and breathing exercises can be fantastic for sleeping. For example, Karin, who regularly came to a yoga class I ran, only used to be able to sleep for two to four hours a night, but after learning some simple breathing and mindfulness activities, she now regularly reports sleeping for seven to eight hours a night.

Mental decline

Another early sign of ageing might be that we feel that our minds don't work as well as they used to. Sometimes this is a normal sign of ageing; however, a slight but noticeable and measurable decline in cognitive abilities, including memory and thinking skills, is known as mild cognitive impairment (MCI). A person with MCI is at increased risk of developing Alzheimer's or another dementia. Long-term studies have shown that 15 to 20 per cent of those aged 65 and older might have an MCI (Alzheimer's Association 2016, n.d.).

A loss in function can be due to the fact that when we age, the number of nerve cells in the brain typically decreases. However, the brain can partly compensate for this loss in several ways:

- As cells are lost, new connections are made between the remaining nerve cells.

- New nerve cells may form in some areas of the brain, even during old age.

This is known as neuroplasticity, which can be defined as the brain's ability to reorganise itself by forming new neural connections throughout life. It occurs when nerve cells in the brain are able to compensate for injury or decline by adjusting their activities in response to changes. This happens when damaged cells grow new parts to reconnect broken links. However, in order to reconnect, the neurons need activity to be stimulated. Unfortunately, for many people, ageing brings a decline in activity (both physical and mental), which makes it difficult to provide this stimulation. Yoga and meditation have been shown to be fantastic for the brain. In fact, studies on long-term meditators have shown increased positive brain activity (Tang, Hölzel and Posner 2005).

Psychiatric conditions such as depression and anxiety

Many people start to feel more anxious and sadder as they get older. This may be the result of stresses caused by personal losses, including of loved ones, health worries and other major life changes, but it can also be the result of physical conditions such as heart disease, neurologic illness, thyroid and other hormone problems.

Incidents of depression may increase as we age due to psychological factors, but also natural body changes associated with ageing may increase a person's risk of experiencing depression. Recent studies suggest that lower concentrations of folate (a type of B vitamin) in the blood and nervous system may contribute to depression, mental impairment and dementia (American Psychological Association n.d.). Many of the foods outlined in the text box on page 49 in Chapter 3 contain high levels of folate.

Feelings of depression and anxiety can also be heightened when we find our vision and hearing becoming poorer, as this may make us feel more vulnerable, less confident and more isolated. Loss in vision and hearing is known as dual-sensory impairment (DSI); studies show between 9 and 21 per cent of adults older than 70 having some degree of DSI (Saunders and Echt 2007).

Many studies show that yoga, meditation and mindfulness have a huge positive impact on anxiety and depression.

Weaker breathing

When we age, the muscles used in breathing, such as the diaphragm and intercostal muscles, tend to weaken. In addition, cell degeneration means that the number of air sacs (alveoli) and capillaries in the lungs also decreases. Thus, slightly less oxygen is absorbed from the air than is breathed in. Deterioration of lung elasticity and capacity can also cause breathing difficulties. As we explore further later, oxygen and deep breathing plays a vital role in our feeling of wellness and our body's ability to repair itself. Yogic breathing exercises (pranayama) are fantastic for improving how we breathe, by encouraging deep and slow breathing, and also for strengthening the muscles involved.

Other common conditions of ageing

As well as general feelings of weakness, mental decline and poor breathing mentioned above, there are many other common conditions related to ageing, and I briefly touch on these before going in to more detail about how yoga can help.

As we age, many people experience disorders of the circulatory system such as hypertension (high blood pressure). This is often due to the decreased sensitivity of the baroreceptors. Baroreceptors are pressure sensors located in the blood vessels of all vertebrate animals. They sense blood pressure and relay this information to the brain. Many factors such as diet, physical activity and genetics can contribute to hypertension. Poor blood circulation and damage to the heart tissues can also be a side effect of many of the diseases mentioned here. Yoga has been shown to reduce blood pressure.

The nervous system is made up of the central nervous system and the peripheral nervous system. It consists of the brain and spinal cord, and all other neural elements including the peripheral nerves and the autonomic nerves. The nervous system can be damaged by a number of factors including trauma, infections and blood flow disruptions. Degenerative disorders of the nervous system include vascular disorders such as stroke, structural disorders such as brain or spinal cord injury, and carpal tunnel syndrome, and degeneration such as Parkinson's disease and Alzheimer's disease, which we address in more detail in the next chapter. I have seen first hand the effect of stroke on my father, how it affected his sight and ability to communicate, and how frustrating this was for him. Yoga has a soothing effect on the nervous system.

The prime function of the immune system is to protect the body against infection, disease and the development of cancer. To support the immune system we need to adopt a healthy lifestyle, manage our stress, exercise and eat a healthy diet. The thymus is responsible for many immune system functions, including the production of T lymphocytes, a type of white blood cell, and other hormones that regulate immune functions.

Low levels of these hormones in the blood are associated with depressed immunity and an increased susceptibility to infection. Typically thymus gland hormone levels will be low in the elderly as the thymus reduces in size as we age. The size of the thymus also reduces in cancer and AIDS patients, and when an individual is exposed to undue stress due to the presence of hormones such as cortisol. As we get older, resilience to deal with stressful situations and our reserve capacity become more important. 'Reserve capacity' is used to describe the body's ability to recover from injury, exertion and disease. This is very important as we get older, as our bodies tend to take longer to get better. Again, yoga, meditation and mindfulness are fantastic for improving the body and mind's ability to deal with stressful situations.

So there is a large number, variety and complexity of common conditions we might suffer from as we age, and more and more people are now living with two or more diseases. When this occurs, medication, or the side effects of medication, may mask symptoms of new diseases and make these difficult to detect. Burdens on medical practitioners' time, and gaps in social care, can also lead to misdiagnosis or poor recovery rates, placing further stress on patients and family members.

It is worthwhile noting that many of the diseases and common conditions mentioned above are either directly, or indirectly, impacted by stress. The ability of yoga and meditation to reduce stress is one of the main ways it works on a therapeutic level, and we explore this in more depth later in this chapter.

Chronological, biological and psychological age

The health of our bodies as we age can be related to both our *chronological age* and *biological age*, as these types of ageing often go together, that is, the physiological state of our bodies mirrors how many years we have been alive. Ageing does have the potential to bring bad health and suffering, and many feel that the deterioration of the body is an inevitable part of getting older. However, the experience of thousands of years of practice of yoga and meditation have revealed many secrets to living a healthier and more fulfilling life.

There are many ways we can separate chronological age from biological age, and I am sure that you will have examples from your friends and family group who live well into their 90s perhaps with no illness, disease and little mental decline. The biological age of our bodies very much depends on how we treat our bodies and the lifestyles we live. Later in this chapter and throughout this book we explore simple methods from yoga and meditation that can help us slow down our biological age.

Psychological age, which is related to mental decline, is both about how we feel mentally, and also our capacity to respond to various changes and events that might happen in our lives. In short, psychological age can be considered a person's adaptive capacity compared to those of the same chronological age. Psychological age is also linked with factors such as how open we are to new experiences, how judgemental we are, and how we cope with both good and bad experiences in life. It is also linked to stress, and how resilient we are to it.

Our psychological age has a huge impact on our biological age in terms of how we treat our bodies, what activities we take part in and how interested we are in our own health. Yoga, as well as addressing our physical bodies, also uses the mind. In my experience people are much happier if they feel that they are growing and learning new skills. Yoga provides this.

SOCIAL AGEING

As well as the physical changes a person goes through, how society views older people is a huge factor in how ageing is perceived. Ageing is approached very differently across different cultures. In many eastern and traditional cultures older people were seen as a valuable part of society. They were the repositories of traditional knowledge and experience, and seen as a vital part of family life. Grandparents would often live with their children, and provide vital help and assistance in childcare and other household tasks. This not only benefited their children, but also the older generation remained engaged in meaningful activities and kept active. For example, in India my cousin lives in a joint family with the grandparents living with their children and grandchildren. My aunt, who is in her mid-70s, thrives on her interactions with her grandchildren, and keeps busy looking after them. This gives my aunt and uncle a sense of purpose, and my cousins really appreciate the help as it enables them to go to work without needing expensive childcare.

Modern western society has changed remarkably in the last hundred years or so – society is much more individualistic, and the extended family is largely a thing of the past. Children often live far away from their parents, and grandparents do not play an active part in their grandchildren's upbringing. Therefore, when some people retire they find that they are negatively affected by a lack of purpose. This doesn't, of course, happen to all people, and many have active and fulfilling retirements. However, for many, retirement brings with it a sense of loneliness, a reduction in physical activity and a corresponding impact on psychological age.

In addition, society often has certain expectations about how people of a certain generation should act. How often do we hear phrases such as 'Why don't you act your age?' or 'You can't teach an old dog new tricks.' This can lead to older people feeling that they are not welcome in certain environments, are not allowed to have fun, or are not expected to keep growing and learning.

In western societies, as life becomes more busy and stressful, older people are often marginalised, lonely and ignored. Societies tend to be more individual and wealth-focused, and I believe that communities and multi-generational friendships have declined. When people reach old age many of their friends and family may have died, and they might lack the transport, independence, confidence or finances to be able to travel and visit the friends they have left. Many might find that the clubs or activities provided (although often by well-meaning volunteers) are patronising, or have no meaning for them. When we have spent a lifetime creating our own lives, and developing individual interests, finding something that appeals to a wide group can be challenging.

Furthermore, social attitudes to diet, health and fitness can also have a huge impact on how people age. For example, in the west a lot of socialising involves eating and drinking, which might counter the positive effects group activity might bring. And many people see exercising as being boring, difficult or a chore.

YOGIC PERSPECTIVES ON AGEING

So far we have discussed various approaches and views on ageing, and how these are so often interlinked. For example, how society views older people can have a huge impact on their confidence and willingness to participate in activities. Eastern cultures are often not so dualistic and do not believe in a separation of mind and body. Additionally, many eastern cultures also promote daily exercise routines that are suitable for all. For example, in China and Thailand many middle-aged and elderly people living in cities perform morning group exercise classes including practices such as Tai Chi. Tai Chi is an ancient Chinese form of martial art and takes many forms, but is often practised for its health benefits, and some forms are considered particularly suitable for older people. These group sessions are often free, suitable for a group and provide an opportunity to meet people at a similar stage in life, to connect and avoid loneliness. In India, many neighbourhoods have gentle yoga sessions which are suitable for the elderly, and often traditional yoga is popular, very accessible and made up of gentle exercises.

People have been performing yoga exercises for thousands of years. However, much of the knowledge about yoga and its benefits were passed down by oral tradition. We have seen above how physical, mental and social elements are all strongly interlinked. If we feel well and have a purpose in life (known in yogic philosophy as dharma), we are more likely to take better care of our health and wellbeing. Instead of the view of health as always having a cause and effect, the yogic view is much more rounded and holistic. It is about bringing the mind, body and breath into better alignment. As the benefits of yoga are many and varied, it is sometimes difficult to test in medical trials. However, in recent years, the practice and idea of using yoga therapeutically has grown. This has resulted in more medical studies showing the benefits of yoga and meditation.

KEY WAYS IN WHICH YOGA WORKS

In this section we explore some examples of how yoga can help with various facets of ageing, including evidence from recent research trials. These are expanded on further in the next chapter, where we outline how yoga can help people living with dementia.

We have seen earlier that yoga works on a number of levels, and is made up of eight different limbs (see page 46), and in this section we draw across all of these practices. However, essential to and underlying all of these is the practice of self-study or self-enquiry, known as svadhyaya. Modern life is increasingly outward-focused as social media results in people seeking to portray a sugar-coated image of themselves online. However, yogic and contemplative practices urge us to be present and to look inwards. This enables us to understand ourselves better and to respond better to early warnings of issues, whether physical, emotional or mental.

Increasing physical strength and energy

The third limb of yoga, asana, is made up of physical positions. The number of these positions ranges greatly, depending on the type of yoga practised, and there are lists of hundreds if not thousands of yogic positions. These can be divided up into limbering exercises, forward and backward bending poses, twists, supine (lying down) positions, inversions (upside-down positions), balancing positions, meditation positions and relaxation poses.

Their variety and the fact that they will take you through a full range of movements provides a great way of exercising and strengthening the whole body. This is opposite to other types of exercise that involve a lot of similar movements and can result in RSI or imbalances in the body, for example, golf, tennis or running. The practice of yoga asana can improve muscle strength and flexibility (Tran *et al.* 2001), and by feeling fitter, we often have more energy.

As mentioned in Chapter 3, yoga also works on the nadis (or energy channels), and it is believed that these are linked to nervous pathways and circulatory systems. Chinese medicine recognises these as meridian lines, and calls the energy chi. Yoga, through coordinated movement and compressing and releasing muscles, helps to clear or cleanse these channels. These movements can increase blood circulation, which in turn has positive effects on the organs, and helps the mind. It is also believed that these movements help stimulate under-used neural pathways, and can therefore help the mind as well as the body.

Improving the mind

People often complain about mental decline as they age. The brain is one of the body's most powerful organs, and uses three times as much oxygen as the muscles. Oxygen is vital to brain function and brain healing. There are various ways of increasing blood flow to the brain including exercising, stretching, inverted positions (or where the legs are above the heart), deep breathing and meditating. Yoga provides all of these.

Yoga, through contemplation, can also provide an internal still place of reference for people living with dementia, where they are not focused on their own anxiety. Daily mindfulness practices can also help people stay in the present moment and not in the past. This is very important as we age, as many people feel sad when thinking about the past and the things they used to be able to do.

Yoga has been proven to help with anger management, depression and anxiety, which can all become more common as we age.

Decreasing stress

We have seen how stress can be a contributing factor to many diseases and conditions, from high blood pressure to cancer. However, in order to understand how yoga and meditation works, we first need to look at how stress affects the body and mind. The nervous system links all of the body's organs and muscles and has a huge impact on many diseases and conditions.

Parasympathetic system   Sympathetic system

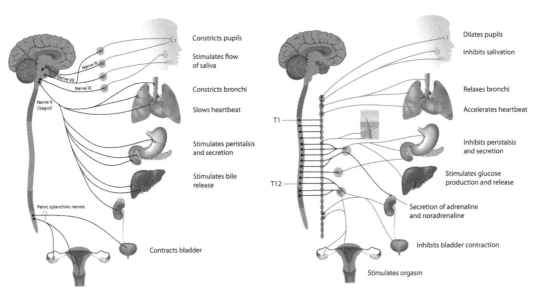

The body has two main divisions of the nervous system – the parasympathetic nervous system (PNS) and the sympathetic nervous system (SNS). The main purpose of the SNS is to stimulate the body's fight or flight response. When we are in a stressful situation the production of hormones such as cortisol activates the SNS and gets the body ready for action, either to fight or flee, hence 'fight or flight'. The heart rate increases, blood flows away from the digestive and reproductive systems, and flows to the muscles. However, for many people, life has become more stressful, resulting in the body being in a constant state of alert. The SNS is also switched on when a person remembers or tells a story about a stressful situation, which is why mental training via relaxation and mindfulness plays such an important part.

The PNS, which is sometimes called the 'rest and digest' system, works to conserve energy as it slows the heart rate, increases intestinal and gland activity, and relaxes sphincter muscles in the gastrointestinal tract. In this state more blood flows to the digestive system and the heart rate lowers, hence 'rest and digest'.

Yoga in particular, through its slow, deep breathing methods, activates PNS. When we are relaxed we breathe slowly and deeply, and conversely, when we breathe slowly and deeply, we become more relaxed. Deep breathing also works on a physical level by increasing the flow of oxygen to the muscles and organs, aiding recovery. Breath work also raises the level of serotonin and lowers the levels of monoamine oxidase that feature in depression, which is common in those living with dementia.

YOGA AND OLDER PEOPLE

So why is yoga particularly suitable for the older generation? The type of yoga in this book is gentle, effective and easy to learn. As well as providing much, much more, yoga can also be considered a form of exercise. It can involve aerobic activity and strength-building exercises, and stretches all the major muscle groups.

The western world often tends to separate the mind and the body, whilst eastern philosophies often see the mind and body as an inseparable entity. We have seen that the interplay of mental and physical age is very important. More and more we see how mental diseases such as anxiety can have a massive impact on our physical bodies, and how our physical wellbeing has a huge impact on our mental state. Yoga, through being a mind-body therapy, takes into account both physical and mental wellbeing.

We all know that exercise is good for our health, no matter how young or old we are. In the UK the National Health Service (NHS) recommends that adults over the age of 65 who have no limiting health conditions should be active daily and do at least 150 minutes of moderate aerobic activity every week, and strength exercises on two or more days a week that work all the major muscle groups.

Falls are a serious problem and are estimated to cost the NHS more than £2.3 billion per year. Postural and balance problems are a key risk in this. Older adults at risk of falls, such as people with weak legs, poor balance and some medical conditions, should do exercises (e.g. yoga, Tai Chi or dancing) to improve their balance and coordination on at least two days a week. However, many people do not meet these guidelines, and in the UK physical inactivity costs the NHS an estimated £1.06 billion a year in direct costs (NICE 2015). The cost of lack of physical activity goes further than pure economic analysis, as being physically fit and active has many emotional as well as physical benefits. In addition, most people living in a residential care environment do not carry out any regular exercise.

I am now going to tell you the story of my grandmother, and I have come to realise that this is a familiar story, as I have heard similar versions of it from many of my clients and their relatives. My grandmother, Dorothea, was fit and active well into her late 80s. She did all her own gardening, household chores, walking to the shops and swimming. However, when she was 89 she had a fall, and had to have a hip replacement. The fall literally knocked the confidence out of her, especially when it came to her physical abilities. At the same time the dementia she was living with became much worse and she became dependent on others for care, eventually moving into a nursing home when caring for her became too much for my mother. The reduction in my grandmother's physical confidence, and related reduction in physical activity, led to a drastic decline in her quality of life. My grandmother became afraid of moving and more fearful. This fear led to anxiety and stress, thereby reducing her body's ability to heal itself.

Finding safe and sustainable types of exercise for older adults that are suitable for those with physical restrictions, such as being at risk of falls, and other pre-existing conditions, is a key challenge for modern society. In addition, an important factor in encouraging people of all ages to exercise is ensuring that the exercise itself is enjoyable and mentally stimulating.

We now go on to look at the many reasons why yoga is so incredibly suitable for older adults.

Overcoming fear

Many older adults who have had falls or feel they are overweight or unfit may lack the confidence to try out new exercise forms. Often potential clients say to me, 'I'm so inflexible, I can't do yoga.' Also, those who encourage older people to exercise may worry about hurting them, especially if they are frail or fearful. Many may believe exercising might be difficult, or have had bad experiences of exercising in the past. People might also be disappointed that they are unable to do the things that they did in the past, or their bodies will not respond in the way they wish. The yoga used in this book and the sequences described provide suitable exercises for all levels and abilities, and modifications are available for all.

One of the key learning points from my research project was the need to ensure we were putting the person or people we are working with at the centre of our decisions. Whether we are starting a yoga practice ourselves, with a family member, a friend or a client, what this means is to start where we and they are today: we need to focus on what we can do, and what we want to do, and use this as a starting point. Personally, I have been surprised at how willing older people are to try new movements and activities. For example, when I first started volunteering in a residential care home, I worked with Reggie. Reggie was in his late 80s and had suffered a stroke that had affected his ability to communicate. He was quite private and tended to keep himself to himself in the home. However, he loved the group yoga classes and reported that they were one of his favourite parts of the week. He also said that they relieved his back pain and that the calmness he felt after the yoga classes helped his speech and communication.

The yoga in this book starts with simple, slow and mindful chair-based exercises that are enjoyable and help to build confidence and reduce fear. They aim to bring back the pleasure people feel in natural movements and the enjoyment of feeling their bodies move. We often see this pleasure in the way children or animals move. When we see a dog getting up from sleeping or a cat stretching we can observe how much they enjoy moving their bodies; for many, when they get to adulthood, they forget this natural enjoyment of movement.

Motivation

Another key aspect is motivation. If older adults have not engaged in any 'formal' exercises or sport in their earlier life, they might not fully appreciate the health and other benefits of regular exercise. Therefore, starting something new might seem like a huge challenge, and many people might think 'what's the point?' However, once they start, older adults often really enjoy the mental and physical stimulation of doing new movements and learning a new skill. And although the effects of yoga increase if practised regularly and over time, most people start to feel the benefits even after one or two sessions. Yoga, with its mixture of dynamic movements and guided relaxations, enables people to go on a journey that often ends in an extremely peaceful state during the relaxation at the end of sessions. This feeling of peace and calm is invaluable, and can help motivate people to continue with the practice.

Accessibility

Another key factor in encouraging people to exercise is accessibility. For many older adults living in the community there might not be a suitable yoga class for their age range. While there has been a huge growth in the numbers of people practising yoga, and yoga teachers, many of these focus on yoga for healthy adults rather than older people or those with physical or mental impairments. Many older adults suffer from loneliness, and practising yoga together can help people find a sense of community. The yoga contained in this book enables people living with dementia, their friends, relatives or carers to be able to practise and benefit together.

CONCLUSION

In this chapter we have discussed many aspects of ageing. As medicine has advanced, infectious diseases have declined; however, as people live longer, they also live more sedentary lives, and as a consequence, lifestyle-related diseases have increased. Yoga, through skilful adaptation and adjustment, can be suitable for all and bring people together. Yoga is an empowering practice, and once people have practised the simple sequences in this book, they can learn to include enjoyable techniques in their daily lives that will improve their health and wellbeing.

CHAPTER 6

WHAT IS DEMENTIA AND HOW CAN YOGA HELP?

In this chapter we explore what dementia is, including different types of dementia, its global prevalence and spread. We also discuss what is known about how dementia affects people, their carers and loved ones, the different stages of dementia, and what we can do to help prevent it.

We then go on to look at how yoga can help those living with dementia. This expands on the previous chapter, and looks at how yoga can help prevent dementia, and also how it can help people living with dementia stay well for longer.

If you are reading this book it is highly likely that you know or work with someone who is living with dementia. Or maybe you have had an early diagnosis, or a family history of dementia, and are looking for appropriate activities to do either by yourself or together with a friend or a relative. Or perhaps you are a yoga teacher or an activities coordinator who is looking for suitable yoga sequences and poses to do with those living with dementia. Regardless, it is highly likely that you will have some understanding of dementia and its impacts. However, as you may be aware, dementia takes on many forms, so here are some basic facts about dementia.

You may already know that dementia has no known cure. However, you might not know that:

- Dementia mainly affects those over the age of 65, although cases of early onset dementia are increasing.

- Symptoms include loss of memory, difficulty performing everyday tasks, language problems, disorientation in time and space, misplacing things, changes in personality including depression, anxiety, anger and loss of initiative.

- One in three US seniors die with dementia (Alzheimer's Association 2016), and many also die from dementia. You might ask how can a person die from dementia. Whilst it is true that many people with late-stage dementia may die of a medical complication, such as pneumonia or another infection, dementia itself can be fatal, for example, from deterioration in the brain.

- Dementia costs the UK economy £23 billion a year, more than cancer and heart disease combined.

- It is estimated that by 2021 one million people will be living with dementia in the UK. Numbers will increase dramatically as the population ages and people live longer.

- A report published by Alzheimer's Research UK in 2015 estimated that one in three people born in 2015 will develop dementia.

Dementia is caused by a variety of brain diseases, most commonly Alzheimer's. These diseases result in the loss of brain cells, and affect the brain's ability to function properly. At the early stages dementia is invisible, and new research shows that in certain genetic types of Alzheimer's disease, the brain starts to show changes 20 years before someone starts to experience symptoms. Therefore, it is never too early to start doing activities to help improve our mental and physical wellbeing.

One of the first signs of dementia can be a problem with memory and thinking. However, as the disease progresses and more cells die, physical functions such as walking, eating and even swallowing can be affected. There are currently no treatments to stop or slow the progression of Alzheimer's disease or other types of dementia, although there are things we can do, including yoga and healthy eating (see the text box on page 49, Chapter 3), to help reduce the risk of developing dementia and to enable us to improve our day-to-day functioning and overall wellbeing.

You probably already know that there is no known cure for dementia. A surgeon cannot simply cut into the brain and fix it. A psychologist cannot identify a cause and set a treatment plan to work through it. It is also important to understand that dementia is not a disease or a specific illness. It is a group of symptoms often wrongly associated with age-related cognitive (mental) decline, and can be related to a number of diseases and conditions. One of the reasons that yoga is so effective is that it treats a number of underlying conditions, in particular, those directly impacted by stress, such as hypertension (high blood pressure). In the section below we explore some common types of dementia and their symptoms.

TYPES OF DEMENTIA

Alzheimer's disease

Alzheimer's disease is one of the most common causes of dementia and accounts for 60–80 per cent of cases. It is estimated that about half of people living with Alzheimer's are also likely to be affected by another form of dementia (see below). When this occurs, this is known as mixed dementia.

Early signs of Alzheimer's include difficulty remembering recent conversations, names or events. Apathy and depression are also common in the early stages. As the disease progresses it can result in communication difficulties, disorientation, confusion, poor judgement, behaviour changes, and towards the later stages, difficulty speaking, swallowing and walking. Alzheimer's is a slowly progressive disease that begins well before symptoms start to appear.

People with Alzheimer's have an accumulation of a type of plaque (a microscopic protein fragment called a beta-amyloid) outside the neurons in their brain, and twisted strands of a protein called tau (tangles) inside their neurons.

Common changes also include a loss of connections among the brain cells responsible for learning, communication and memory. These connections transmit information from cell to cell. The body's immune system also responds by triggering inflammation, which has been shown to be reduced by yoga (Ross and Thomas 2010). These changes are eventually accompanied by the damage and death of neurons and brain tissue shrinkage (Alzheimer's Association 2015).

Vascular dementia

Vascular dementia is a form of dementia caused by a stroke or multiple strokes (known in medical terminology as infarcts). This type of dementia accounts for only approximately 10 per cent of cases as a sole cause. However, many older individuals with other forms of dementia will have evidence of vascular dementia as well, that is, mixed dementia. Early signs of vascular dementia include poor judgement and decision-making abilities, as opposed to memory loss. Vascular dementia occurs most often from blood vessel blockage or damage leading to strokes (infarcts) or bleeding in the brain. The location, number and size of these bleeds can vary dramatically and will affect whether they will result in dementia and how individual physical and mental abilities will be affected. It is believed that learning new skills, such as yoga, that require focused concentration helps the mind to repair itself, a process known as neuroplasticity.

Dementia with Lewy bodies

Lewy bodies are formed of abnormal clumps of a protein called alpha-synuclein that accumulates in neurons. Whilst alpha-synuclein is a commonly forming protein in the brain, when it forms into Lewy bodies it is believed that these displace other cell components. Alpha-synuclein also aggregates in the brains of people with Parkinson's disease. People with dementia with Lewy bodies often find that their mental abilities are impaired, whereas with Parkinson's disease, the Lewy bodies affect the part of the brain that controls movement.

Other types of dementia

Another common type of dementia especially amongst those under 65 is *frontotemporal lobar degeneration* (FTLD). This category includes a number of different diseases. It affects nerve cells in the front and side regions of the brain (frontal and temporal lobes), and these regions become shrunken. In addition, upper layers of the brain become soft and spongy. Early symptoms of this type of dementia include marked changes in personality and behaviour, and difficulties speaking and comprehending. Unlike Alzheimer's disease memory is typically spared in the early stage of disease. FTLD is the second most common degenerative dementia in the younger (around 60) age group.

Other types of dementia include *Parkinson's disease*, which mainly involves problems with control of movements but can later result in dementia. *Creutzfeldt-Jakob disease* is a rare and fatal disorder that impairs memory and coordination and causes behaviour changes. It is the result of a misfolded protein that causes other proteins in the brain to misfold and malfunction. It may be hereditary, sporadic or caused by an infection. Another form of dementia, called *normal pressure hydrocephalus*, accounts for less than 5 per cent of cases. A build-up of fluid on the brain causes this type of dementia. Its symptoms include difficulty with walking, memory loss and inability to control urination. People with a history of brain haemorrhage and meningitis are at increased risk of this.

It is now thought that over half of those with dementia have some form of *mixed dementia* (evidence of more than one cause of dementia). The fact that so many people have mixed dementia, and that there are so many types of dementia, makes it a very difficult disease to predict or cure. However, yoga offers us the opportunity to take a holistic view of our health and to do things that benefit the whole body and mind, which in turn has positive benefits for all types of dementia.

A DIAGNOSIS OF DEMENTIA

There is no one test to determine if someone has dementia. Instead, to make a diagnosis doctors use a careful medical history, a physical examination, laboratory tests and note changes in thinking, day-to-day function and behaviour associated with each type of dementia. However, studies reveal many cases of delayed and/or undocumented diagnosis of dementia among primary care providers. This can be for a variety of reasons, including lack of information, presence of other diseases, lack of resources, perceived lack of treatment options or a belief that little or nothing can be done for patients with dementia.

There are also ethical questions about whether a person wants to know about their diagnosis of dementia. Lots of people and their loved ones believe it would be better not to know. The fact that dementia can often be combined with loneliness, depression and other illnesses means that doctors might be reluctant to disclose someone's diagnosis. Personally, although I can understand the reluctance sometimes to diagnose dementia, I find it quite worrying, as it adds to the culture of 'burying your head in the sand', negativity and shame that exists around dementia.

Being diagnosed with dementia is challenging, not just for the person receiving the diagnosis, but also for their friends and relatives and the person giving the diagnosis. It challenges doctors' professional skills and also raises difficult questions about a person's best interests, independence and dignity. However, studies have shown that many people would prefer to receive an honest diagnosis of their condition. This enables people, their carers and families to plan, and also to make appropriate changes and adaptations. As discussed in Chapter 3, key tenets of yoga are satya (truthfulness) and svadhyaya (self-study), and these point to the need to be honest about our, or our relatives or friends', condition. The examples below show some of the benefits of early diagnosis.

David and Alzheimer's

David was a resident I worked with at the first care home I started teaching yoga at. He started noticing that he had begun to forget things in his mid-70s and, after discussing with his doctor and undergoing a number of tests, he was diagnosed with Alzheimer's disease. He told his family and close friends, and together they read all they could about the disease, and researched coping strategies. They established ways of ensuring that David kept active and focused on doing the things he wanted to do and remember. David's wife made handy laminated notes to help David with simple tasks.

David's children helped him make a memory book that included some fantastic stories about his experiences of being evacuated from London during the war. As David's family knew about David's diagnosis, they made allowances for him when he got frustrated, angry or felt down. While David was still in the early stages he discussed his wishes with his family so they knew what he wanted as his disease progressed. David was later transferred to a care home when it was too much for his family to care for him at home. David had been clear that he did not want to be a burden on his family, and these were his wishes. Whilst at the home, David's family helped him complete his memory book. Although David passed away from complications due to his disease when he was in his late 80s, his family felt that he had had the best care possible, and he had been able to keep active and moving for as long as he could by taking part in the yoga classes. They have a fantastic record of his memories to cherish and share.

June's diagnosis

I met June at a later project I was working on. In June's case she also noticed that she was getting more forgetful in her early 70s, but put this down to normal ageing, and did not inform any of her family or discuss things with her doctor. As her symptoms progressed she became increasingly more confused and scared. She began to lash out at her loved ones, who then felt she was pushing them away. Although her family became increasingly worried about her, they did not want to broach the subject with her. Later June had a fall at home and was transferred to hospital, and then into a home, where her condition deteriorated. June later joined in some of my yoga classes, which she enjoyed. Talking to her family after one of the sessions they said they felt sad that they hadn't known about her dementia earlier, and experienced a lot of regret that they had not been able to spend more time with her when she was able to understand more.

People and society in general are much more comfortable talking about physical illnesses than talking about diseases that affect the mind. This might be because they find these types of diseases scary and confusing. However, as more and more people will develop dementia each year, we need to get better about talking about the condition. Personally, I have a higher risk of developing dementia as family history is a risk factor. It is one of my sincere hopes that in the future there will be much better communication and discussions about the disease.

STAGES OF DEMENTIA

The next part of this chapter looks at the stages of dementia. As there is no cure for dementia; the symptoms will increase over time, although this can vary greatly; for example, on average a person with Alzheimer's disease will live for four to eight years after diagnosis. However, some people might live for as long as 20 years. For many people (and their families) living with Alzheimer's or another form of dementia, the uncertainty of not knowing what will happen to them or how quickly is very unsettling. It can also make planning for care and other financial planning very difficult, leading to further stress and anxiety.

Dementia has been divided into a number of stages depending on which model you use. However, it is important to recognise that as the progression of the disease varies so much, these stages are only guidelines and useful for a planning/communication point of view. One of the most common scales is called the Global Deterioration Scale for Assessment of Primary Degenerative Dementia. While this divides the disease progression into seven stages depending on the effects on the mind, it is more common to refer to three stages of dementia. These stages and their common symptoms are explained below.

This book contains yoga poses and exercises for all stages of dementia. These can help alleviate the symptoms and help the person feel well in the moment. At the early/mid-stage, they can be done independently; however, at the late stage, people will need assistance and they are best done together with a carer, family member or loved one. Although designed for those living with dementia, the exercises will benefit all those who are doing them, including carers and family members. In fact, the manager of a care home where these exercises were introduced commented that the overall wellbeing on the whole of the dementia unit improved as part of the yoga project.

Early-stage dementia

At the early stage of dementia a person might be able to function independently. They may be able to drive and take part in normal social activities. However, they may find they are having memory lapses, or forget familiar words or the location of everyday objects. Family members or friends might begin to notice difficulties. Common symptoms include forgetting something they have just read, losing something, increased trouble planning or organising, and problems coming up with the right word or name of something.

This book has a number of sequences for early-stage dementia, in particular, those in Chapter 9, which help maintain cognitive functioning. They involve coordinated movements that help to stimulate the brain, and strengthening exercises to keep the body strong, release tension and build physical confidence.

Mid-stage dementia

Mid-stage or moderate dementia is typically the longest stage and can last for many years. At this stage damage to the nerves might make it difficult for the person to express thoughts or perform routine tasks. The person might confuse words, get angry or frustrated and/or act in unexpected ways. Other noticeable symptoms may include forgetfulness of events, or about their personal history, being withdrawn or depressed, or being unable to remember their own address or telephone number. The person might need help choosing appropriate clothes for the time of year, or get confused about what day it is; there might also be an increased risk of becoming lost or wandering. Some people have personality or behaviour changes including suspiciousness, delusion or compulsive behaviour.

The yoga for mid-stage dementia contained in this book focuses on exercises that help release energy and frustration, keep the body supple and movements that help with anger management. Some examples of yoga for mid-stage dementia can be found in Chapters 8, 10 and 11.

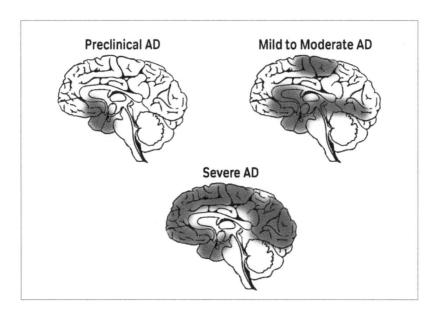

Late-stage dementia

In the late or advanced stage of dementia the person loses the ability to respond to their environment, to hold a conversation and eventually to control their movements. Drastic personality changes might occur as memory and cognitive skills deteriorate.

At this stage the person might need around-the-clock assistance with daily personal care. They might lose awareness of recent experiences as well as of their surroundings. The person might also experience changes in physical abilities including being able to walk, sit, and eventually swallow. They might also be vulnerable to infections, especially pneumonia.

The yoga sequences for this stage include exercises that can be done with a loved one or carer to keep as much mobility as possible, relaxing exercises and exercises to help the person feel connected and loved. This book also includes some very simple exercises that can be done lying down, and Chapter 14 is dedicated to gentle practice that can be done with those with late-stage dementia.

RISK FACTORS FOR DEMENTIA

The exact causes of dementia can be varied, and there is no one factor that causes it (except in rare genetic cases; see below). This is one of the reasons it is so difficult to find a cure. Also, understanding exactly how the human brain works is still a great mystery to the scientific world, as the human brain is one of the world's more complex objects. However, despite this, a number of risk factors for dementia have been found.

The most prominent is age, and the older we are, the more likely we are to get Alzheimer's disease; for example, nearly one in three people over the age of 85 has Alzheimer's. The reason why the risks increase so dramatically as we grow older is one of the mysteries of Alzheimer's.

Another key risk is if we have a family history of dementia, and if we have a brother, sister or parent with Alzheimer's, we are more likely to develop the disease. There are two types of genes involved in Alzheimer's. One is a risk gene, which means that there is a higher risk of developing the illness. The other, which is found in a small number of family groups, is a deterministic gene. These cases are when all family members will get the disease, and often it will start to appear in in those under 60 but can start appearing when someone is in their 30s or 40s. These cases are very rare and only account for about 5 per cent of all cases worldwide. These genetic cases can also help scientists investigate the disease and trial potential cures.

REDUCING THE RISK

You might be reading this book as a carer or relative of someone who is living with dementia, and perhaps you are wondering if there are ways of reducing your risk of developing dementia. The good news is, yes, there are things that you can do that will help you increase your wellbeing across your life course.

It is believed that overall healthy ageing will help to decrease the risk of developing dementia. So, using yoga or other methods to try to keep to a healthy weight, avoiding tobacco and excess alcohol will all lessen your risk. Also, staying socially connected and doing exercises that stimulate both the body and mind are very important for keeping healthy. Yoga can help build strength and endurance, and tests have shown that an eight-week yoga programme resulted in a 31 per cent increase in students' muscular strength and a 57 per cent increase in muscle endurance (Tran *et al.* 2001).

Yogic philosophy promotes the idea of a strong connection between the brain and the heart. In early stages of human development in the womb the heart develops first and the head and heart emerge from the same area of tissue. Growing medical evidence links brain health to heart health. This makes complete sense as the brain is supplied by one of the richest networks of blood vessels. About 20–25 per cent of blood from each heartbeat goes to the brain, and the brain uses at least 20 per cent of the nutrients and oxygen carried by the blood. The risk of developing vascular dementia and Alzheimer's disease seems to increase with conditions that damage the heart or blood vessels including stroke, diabetes and high cholesterol. We have seen that these are all negatively affected by stress. In addition, the plaques and tangles present in dementia cases are more likely to cause symptoms if the brain's blood vessels have also been damaged, for example, by a stroke.

There is a strong link between head trauma and risk of developing Alzheimer's disease. Therefore, anything you can do to reduce the risk of head injury is important. This includes normal risk-reducing behaviour, such as wearing a seatbelt or a helmet when participating in sports, but also, as we get older, it is important to take steps to reduce the risk of falls. Yoga can help by improving balance, coordination and core strength.

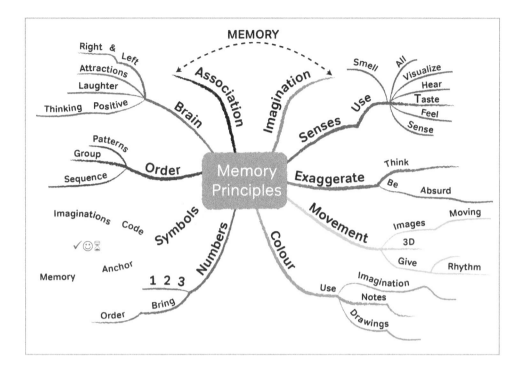

BENEFITS OF YOGA FOR DEMENTIA

In my personal experience of more than 20 years practising and teaching yoga, people respond best, and are more likely to commit to a practice, when they know what the benefits are. We now look at the benefits of yoga for those living with dementia, how these work and relevant recent studies.

The primary aim of any treatment of dementia is to tackle the symptoms, and to provide the patient with the best possible quality of life. This is the aim of the sequences in this book. In the pilot project I led, and in many other reputable studies, there have been many successes for clients living with dementia and the symptoms related to it. My research showed that clients appeared more awake, alert and happy after completing many of the sequences in the book. In addition, clients were able to remember some of the sequences and their moods improved. Yoga for Dementia is innovative and ground-breaking, and I believe that, as more people living with dementia practise yoga, we will begin to see further benefits.

In 2016 a team at UCLA found that a three-month course of yoga and meditation practice helped minimise the cognitive (mental) and emotional problems that often precede Alzheimer's disease and other forms of dementia (Eyre *et al.* 2016). They found that the yoga exercise, which took just 12 minutes each day, was more effective than the memory enhancement exercises, which had been considered the gold standard for managing mild cognitive impairment (MCI). This yoga secret is shared in Chapter 9, which also contains other sequences and exercises to help with early stages of dementia and cognitive impairment.

Depression and dementia are often found together, which is hardly a surprise, as in the early stages of dementia, people might feel confused and bewildered by what is happening to them. The Alzheimer's Association estimates that 20–40 per cent of people with Alzheimer's have significant depression. Yoga has been proven to benefit depression and other neuropsychiatric disorders, and many studies have shown this (e.g. Balasubramaniam, Telles and Doraiswamy 2012). In particular, recent studies have shown that yogic breathing can have a significant impact on depression through its role in taming the stress response. The secret is that yogic breathing helps to switch on the parasympathetic nervous system (PNS), which helps to slow the heart rate, and increase the production of feel-good hormones. Many of the sequences within this book contain targeted breathing exercises and other movements to help with depression. Studies have shown that the same yoga meditation programme mentioned above was also associated with positive changes in mood, anxiety and improved brain blood flow.

In addition, meditation and yoga have anti-ageing effects, and people who meditate have a younger, healthier-looking brain (Ornish *et al.* 2013). They also have more brain blood flow when at rest.

Those living with dementia might also show signs of anger, anxiety or aggression, which may be due to a number of factors such as physical discomfort, environmental factors or poor communication skills. The Alzheimer's Association recommends involving a person in suitable activities, and finding an outlet for a person's anger as a way of dealing with aggression. Yoga and mindfulness-based practices have been shown to reduce feelings of anger, and anxiety amongst various population groups. Chapter 10 is devoted to anger management techniques.

When a person experiences stress for the first time, the body has a physical reaction to that stress, called the 'fight or flight' response (see page 90, Chapter 5). However, when the person retells or remembers the stressful incident, again, the body has the same physical reactions. Therefore, the body does not distinguish between the 'real' incident and the retelling of the incident. Stress and anxiety and their effects on the body are therefore often exacerbated by obsessive repetitive thoughts and worries that tend to increase as we age. Yoga that combines meditation, mindfulness and physical awareness helps a person remain in the here and now. If you have dementia (or have a family member or care for someone with this diagnosis) it is, of course, natural to worry; however, it is important that this does not take over. It is also important not to spend too much time dwelling on the past and what that person could do. The yoga in this book helps us to be in the present and enjoy our lives, no matter what our stage of diagnosis is.

Many people living with dementia also become disorientated and lose their spatial awareness, which is about how we locate our body in space. It is estimated that more than one-third of patients with Alzheimer's have disabling visual-spatial disorientation that interferes with safe driving and independent living (Parnetti and Calabresi 2006). Yoga can help improve awareness of where the body is located in space through bodily awareness techniques. The pushing away the clouds exercise (see page 70, Chapter 4) is particularly good for locating our bodies in space.

MEDITATION

This book combines physical yoga with simple meditation and guided relaxation exercises. Many people who have not tried meditation might find the idea of meditation difficult or unappealing. Meditation is often misunderstood, and many people believe it is about emptying the mind, or sitting for hours on end in an uncomfortable position. Meditation is, in fact, a very simple practice of watching the thoughts, and there are many easy meditation and awareness techniques that are suitable for all. These are found throughout this book, for example, the journey of awareness practice (see page 131, Chapter 8). There is more and more research about the benefits of meditation, and I have outlined some of this below:

- *Regular yoga and meditation practitioners have less atrophy (wastage)* in the hippocampus (the part of the brain thought to be responsible for emotion, memory and the autonomic nervous system), which appears shrunken in people with Alzheimer's disease.

- *Meditation* increases protective tissues *in our brains.*

- *Meditation can help older people feel less isolated.*

- There is a high correlation between perceived stress and Alzheimer's. *Meditation helps participants feel calmer*, lessening perceived stress.

- *Meditation also reduces the stress hormone cortisol,* which has been known to increase the risk of developing dementia.

- *Meditation increases cortical thickness (a measure of the thickness of the important part of the brain) and grey matter*, which slows the ageing rate of the brain. Cortical thickness has been associated with decision-making and memory.

Researchers attribute the positive 'brain fitness' effects of mindful exercise to several factors, including its abilities to reduce stress and inflammation, improve mood and resilience, and enhance production of brain-derived neurotrophic growth factor, a protein that stimulates connections between neurons and kick-starts telomerase activity, replacing lost or damaged genetic material (Eyre *et al.* 2016).

Different meditation techniques have also been shown to create differences in brain blood flow and activation of distinct important areas of the brain. These changes correlate with the depth of meditation, spiritual connectedness and stress reduction.

CARING FOR THE CARERS

Having been a full-time live-in carer for my father, and also being involved when my mother cared for my grandmother in her mid-stage of dementia, I have experienced first hand how stressful and worrying caring for someone with dementia can be. In order to deliver effective dementia care, carers and family members also need to be cared for. More and more we are seeing the stress and burdens of dementia on family caregivers. Yoga and meditation has been shown by a team of researchers (Pomykala *et al.* 2012) also to provide better mental health for dementia caregivers. Benefits include:

- High levels of improvement in mental health and depression were seen amongst highly stressed family dementia caregivers.

- The meditation participants also scored higher in memory tests.

- There was also the largest ever increase in the enzyme telomerase, which is responsible for maintaining telomere length (telomeres are the end of chromosomes that influence our longevity, health and cognitive function).

- Brain function in distressed caregivers improved in significant areas.

The short pilot study by Pomykala *et al.* (2012) shows that caregivers can also benefit from the practices in this book. Many yoga and meditation practices promote the idea of unity and connectedness, and it makes me happy to know that by doing these practices to help others, we are also helping ourselves.

Here is a great exercise we can do as carers, to help us and those we care for.

METTĀ, DEVELOPING LOVING-KINDNESS

Mettā meditation is a popular meditation that helps us develop our love and compassion. Often in today's world, when are exposed to so much suffering on the news and violence on TV, we become desensitised to suffering. Mettā (Pali) or maitrī (Sanskrit) is an ancient word meaning friendliness, benevolence, loving-kindness, good will, an active interest in others and non-violence. It is a meditation practice that helps us cultivate this loving-kindness and compassion for others. Mettā practice is great for people living with dementia, as the instructions are quite repetitive, so if someone forgets where they are in the meditation part way through, it doesn't matter.

Compassion is the ability to understand and relate to others, particularly when others are suffering. While humans are united in their search for happiness, we will all experience some suffering through our lives. Compassion is about recognising that which unites us as humans – a search for happiness and freedom from suffering. Developing compassion towards others including strangers has strong links to our mental health and wellbeing. It helps us feel socially connected to everyone, which is something that dementia can take away; it also helps us maintain a positive outlook on life. Research by psychologist Barbara Fredrickson found that loving-kindness meditation can increase our experiences of emotions such as contentment, hope, gratitude, joy, love and interest (Fredrickson et al. 2008).

To do this exercise, sit or lie down in a comfortable position. You can ask someone to read the instructions to you, or you can do this exercise with one other person or a group. Once you have learned the basic instructions, practise yourself without guidance.

First, bring yourself to mind. Visualise all your good points, and the bits about yourself that you do not like so much. Visualise your physical body, your personality and your voice. Visualise the full uniqueness of you. Next, with an image of yourself in your mind, say these words three times in your mind whilst at the same time feeling the associated feelings and any emotions arising: 'I wish myself love, kindness and freedom from suffering.' As you say the words in your mind, see if you can really hear each word, and focus on the feelings that arise inside you. Try to really extend those feelings to yourself.

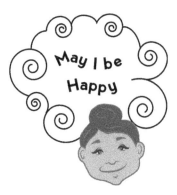

Next, imagine someone or a sentient being you really love. It could be a loved one, friend or favourite pet... Bring that being to mind, visualising them in all their technicolor glory. With the image of them in your mind, say the words to yourself: 'I wish you love, kindness and freedom from suffering', and as you are saying the words, visualise sending that energy and those feelings towards that person...

Next, choose a person you feel quite indifferent to. It could be a person you see on a commute, a work colleague you don't know so well or a client you are not that familiar with. Bring that person to mind and then repeat the same words in your mind. Cultivate the same set of feelings. Try to notice if it feels different from when you were offering the words to someone you love.

Next, choose someone or a situation you know needs healing. It could be an individual, a family conflict or a global situation. Bring that situation or person to mind. You could visualise an iconic image of a conflict, or a symbol that represents it for you. Again, with the situation in mind, say the same words and cultivate the same feelings of love, kindness and freedom from suffering, sending it to that person or situation.

To finish, bring the attention again once more back to yourself. Cultivate the same feelings and compassion for yourself.

As an additional part of the exercise, once you have practised the first stages a few times and are familiar with it, you can add a slightly more difficult stage. Visualise someone you do not like or are having difficulties with. It could be a colleague, client, family member or anyone you have had a bad relationship with. Try to understand that even if we feel we have been wronged, we are unlikely to know the full set of circumstances that led the person to behave in in the way they did.

Bring that person to mind and then, with a mental image of the person in your mind space, say the words clearly to yourself: 'I extend to you love, kindness and freedom from suffering', and try to cultivate the same feeling for that person. Cultivating feelings of compassion for someone we are not on good terms with can be difficult, but just try to do the best you can, and as with any of the exercises in this book, practice makes perfect.

PHYSICAL CONSTRAINTS

Those living with dementia, particularly towards the later stages of the disease, might have some common physical attributes/constraints. These are often combined with other age-related physical disabilities, for example, frailty, balance issues etc. When creating sequences for patients/clients with dementia it is important to consider all of these physical characteristics. Even though not all people living with dementia are chair-bound, and in fact many are very active, many of the sequences are designed to be done from a seated position. A number of more challenging standing sequences are provided for those who are more physically able and in the earlier stages of dementia. Also included in this book are some sequences that can be done from lying down, which will help with later stages of dementia.

The sequences within this book can improve the quality of life and general sense of wellbeing of the person through physical improvements to their body as well as the aforementioned cognitive benefits. Yoga provides a highly suitable form of exercise, and this book contains sequences and exercises for all stages of dementia. These provide strength to muscles where there was little before, help a person develop confidence in movements, and can help with bonding and social interaction, which can allow the person to be more active socially, outside of the yoga sessions.

Yoga may alleviate aches and pains and reduce the risk of future injury, by strengthening and increasing the elasticity of the muscles. Yoga can help to increase a person's balance and reduce falls. But far more importantly, once an elderly person suffers a significant injury with an extended recovery time, such as a pelvic injury, they often enter a rapid decline and never really truly recover, as was the case with my grandmother. This is linked to the massive decrease in their mobility, quality of life and general willingness to fight on.

All that is required to utilise this book, and to achieve positive benefits, is an open mind and a willingness to try those sequences that are suitable for you or those you care for. If you are unsure about any of the sequences in this book, do check out the example sequences contained in the accompanying short videos, which can be accessed at www.jkp.com/voucher using the code PLAHAYYOGA. Also, although the sequences have seriously good benefits, they are also meant to be fun! You must simply ensure you pay attention to all aspects of the sequences, in particular the breathing, meditation and relaxation exercises.

CONCLUSION

In this chapter we have explored what dementia is and the different types of dementia. We also look at the stages of dementia and cognitive decline. I discuss the important of early diagnosis as although the dementia itself might be untreatable, it is often accompanied by reversible conditions. These accompanying conditions might be able to be treated which could help improve brain function and reduce symptoms. An early diagnosis also helps people to increase activities to slow disease progression, understand what is happening to them and plan ahead. We look at the different ways yoga and meditation can help those who are living with dementia and their carers. I also introduce a wonderful exercise to help us develop compassion and loving kindness.

CHAPTER 7

RUNNING YOGA SESSIONS FOR PEOPLE LIVING WITH DEMENTIA

Yoga is a useful and life-affirming practice, and this chapter begins to explore what you will need prior to beginning to use it to enjoy the moment, be spontaneous and make the best of our varying moods. I address what physical and mental tools you will need prior to starting a practice, and small things you can do in the beginning to help make your practice more successful, or that of those you are working with.

If you yourself have had a diagnosis of dementia, or are worried about cognitive impairment (for example, memory and mental decline), the sequences in Chapter 9 are challenging and motivating. These are practices that you can do yourself or with a friend or relative. They will help stimulate your mind, your body and your senses. The kirtan kriya (singing practice) (see page 159, Chapter 9) in particular has been shown to be better than standard mind exercises in reducing cognitive decline (Eyre *et al.* 2016).

If you are working in a community group or nursing home, I provide detailed instructions on how to run a gentle therapeutic yoga session for individuals or groups of clients. If you are worried about leading a yoga-based session, I provide practical tips throughout this book for how to build your own teaching skills with exercises to build your own awareness.

Running yoga sessions with a family member brings challenges. From my own experience I know that in family relations we often fall into set habits, and it is sometimes difficult to break these. I provide some tips on how to run a fun session with your loved one. These will help you live moment to moment. Many of the exercises are also useful for dealing with issues such as anger, sadness or challenging behaviour. Tried and tested approaches are provided for integrating these practices into your loved one's daily life.

Many of the sequences and exercises within this book also show how you can take some time out to 'care for the carer', which is an extremely important place to start.

BASICS FOR TEACHING OR LEARNING YOGA

We have already explored the basic theory of what yoga is, including some of the founding principles, such as the inward codes of conduct (yama) and the outward codes of conduct (niyama). The eight limbs (see Chapter 3) are important for how we decide to practise (and teach) yoga. While many modern yoga practices are primarily concerned with asanas (physical poses), for those living with dementia, the other seven limbs are equally, if not more, important. In previous chapters we have explored the importance of breathing techniques (pranayama) in health. We have also explained how focused concentration (dhyana) helps to rebuild the pathways in the mind.

Another important aspect of yoga is the concept of dharma, which is sometimes wrongly translated as 'duty'. A more accurate description could be 'right action' or 'right path'. Finding your dharma is very much about being in the moment, acceptance and flow. If you are reading this book, you have already committed to taking better care of yourself, a loved one, or someone you work with. At this moment this is your dharma – to care for a precious human life. This work is one of the most important things we can do in life. When a person comes to the end of their life, they do not often regret not working harder, or making more money. What people often regret is not spending more time with their loved ones. In my case, even though I was my father's main carer for a number of years before he died, I still regret not spending more time with him, or being more present with him. I also regret not spending more time with my grandmother before she lost much of her memory and communication skills. I regret the lost stories and memories that were never captured or made. This book is my offering for you, and your loved ones, to be able to experience more peace and more joy right now.

Now you might be saying to yourself, 'Well, how can I possibly lead yoga sessions, having hardly done any myself, or not really knowing much about it?' Let me reassure you: the yogic practices contained in this book, whilst coming from ancient sources, have been carefully adapted to be simple and easy to instruct. As noted in Chapter 1, there are many different types of yoga and there is constant innovation in this field. Modern yoga teachers have adapted yoga positions from ancient practices to suit modern bodies and lifestyles. So, I hear you ask, 'Is yoga made up?' In a sense, yoga is made up, as the initial founders of yoga would have used their own bodies as testing beds. These would have been developed through trial and error, as they still are today. The practices within this book will give you the foundations to be able to design and adapt a practice that is suitable for you or your loved one. A particular point to remember is that whether we have a diagnosis of dementia or not, all of us are individuals. For example, Joan, who I worked with on my project, was a dancer and had been used to doing a lot of physical movements throughout her life. Despite the fact she was living with the mid-stage of dementia, she had a lot of energy and was able to do the more active sequences, such as those in Chapter 8. On the other hand, Henry, even though he was living with the early stages of dementia, had not been so active in his life, and therefore preferred more gentle movements such as those in Chapter 11.

We need to recognise all people will have good and bad days, both physically and mentally. Some days they will want to move more and other days they might want to do less. It is therefore important to work with the person as they are, and to focus on what they can do rather than what they cannot do. Even though someone living with dementia might have lost some of their communication abilities, we need to respect their rights as an individual to have preferences, and to be able to make choices.

If you are using this book for yourself, the first thing we need to explore is what your motivations are for learning yoga. Maybe you may have received an early diagnosis of Alzheimer's disease, or are worried that your mind does not seem to be as sharp as it used to be. Maybe you are seeking a challenging practice to stimulate both body and mind. If this is the case, you have come to the right place.

If you are practising yourself, you may also have some of the complications mentioned in Chapter 5. If this is the case, as always, it is best to speak to your doctor about your intention to start a gentle yoga practice.

MOTIVATIONS FOR TEACHING OR LEARNING

Whenever people are worried about health issues, they are often scared and therefore vulnerable. It is quite common at this point in people's lives for them to be exploited, perhaps by someone offering miraculous cures, or someone selling expensive vitamins or other 'get well quick' fixes. The techniques in this book do not offer to cure dementia, but what they do offer is a way to live in the present moment, with more joy and more happiness.

In Chapter 3 we looked at the eight limbs of yoga. One of these is ahimsa, which means non-violence – this can relate to both physical and mental violence. Physical violence is often easy to understand; however, mental violence can be subtle and is often self-inflicted. For example, we are much more likely to be judgemental towards ourselves and say things like, 'How could I have done that?' or 'How could I have been so stupid?' On the other hand, we might say, 'Oh, don't worry, it doesn't matter' to a loved one who made the same mistake.

This 'being our own worst enemy' or 'self-sabotage' behaviour is common (particularly in the early stages of dementia), destructive, and leads to more pessimism. This is an extremely important point because if you are practising yourself, you might find yourself getting frustrated and feeling disappointed for not being able to do the things you used to be able to do, or for forgetting things. You might also have doubts that you will be able to perform the exercises or remember them. In this case it is important to work on developing self-compassion, and an exercise for this, mettā, is outlined on page 109 (Chapter 6). This will help you to be kind and loving to yourself.

As mentioned in the Introduction, whether you are practising by yourself or with others, it is a good idea to use a notebook so you can record what you have practised and any observations about the impacts of the practice. For example, it is helpful to record the exercises you have tried and how you felt both physically, mentally and emotionally afterwards. A notebook can also help you track longer-term changes.

If you are helping another person practise yoga, ahimsa (non-harming) is very important. Many people living with dementia may also have another illness or disease, may be frail or have a lower pain tolerance than they are used to. They might be less able to communicate how they are feeling, and their wishes. I believe it is important for those who know the person living with dementia to be the ones doing the practices with them. However, if you are a yoga teacher running sessions in a residential care setting, I recommend having one or two carers who know the clients joining in the class. No matter who is giving the class, or doing the practice, it is extremely important to start slowly and gently, maybe just by selecting a few of the simple movements from the basic sequence outlined in Chapter 8. Give these movements a try for 10–15 minutes, and then check in with how you or the people you are working with are feeling. Get some feedback about how they were the rest of the day, and then continue building up the sequence little by little, to ensure you are practising in a way that does no harm.

CARING FOR THE CARER

Care work is often exhausting, stressful and for many non-family carers, it is low-paid with high staff turnover. One of the benefits of yoga is that as well as supporting the person living with dementia, it can also support their carers. The practices within this book provide practical ways of dealing with stress and anxiety, and ways to promote better sleep (such as the yoga nidra exercise on page 234, Chapter 14). Other practices are fantastic for the shoulders, neck and back (such as the shoulder-opening sequence on page 147, Chapter 8), and many of the care staff who were working with me on my project reported a reduction in aches, pains and feelings of stiffness.

People living with dementia often respond on a sensory level, rather than just following verbal instructions. For example, they will note body language or tone of voice. Therefore, it is very important to review your own emotional state before beginning to practise with others. If you are a carer who is planning on using the yoga practices in this book with your family member or clients, I suggest your first try out the exercise you intend to teach and see how it affects you. Whatever you do, do not attempt to do the exercises when you are feeling stressed or anxious, as these feelings are highly likely to be picked up by the person you are caring for. Instead, I recommend doing the journey of awareness exercise outlined on page 131, Chapter 8. This is a fantastic exercise and can be done in as little as 5 minutes. So if you need to, before you begin to practise yoga, give this exercise a try as it will help you feel grounded and ready for the session.

BEFORE YOU BEGIN

Now you might already know a lot about yoga, dementia and other common illnesses, and have skipped forward to this section in your eagerness to get started. This is fine and it is fantastic that you are ready to start. However, I strongly advise you take a moment to review the eight limbs of yoga outlined in Chapter 3, as this lays the foundation of the practices presented in this book.

What you will need

The great thing about true yoga is that it does not require much to practise. Part of its beauty is in its simplicity, and the fact that it can be done anywhere. However, a few easy-to-find things will help aid our practice.

For all practices it is recommended that you, or those you are practising with, wear loose-fitting and comfortable clothing. No special yoga wear is needed, although it is nice to have a few layers, or a shawl, as it is likely your body temperature will vary throughout the sequences. Ideally comfortable shoes, slippers or warm socks that can be easily taken off should be worn. This is to enable us to be able to access the toes and work with the feet. However, if you have a large group, sometimes taking off shoes is impractical, in which case loose-fitting shoes can remain on. For some of the standing sequences either bare feet or shoes with a grip should be worn to minimise the risk of falling.

The sequences in this book are divided into a number of separate sections including introductory sequences for all, challenging and stimulating practices for those who are living with early-stage dementia, practices for anger management, simple and calming sequences for those at mid-stage, and those at a late stage who are looking for simple and enjoyable practices. However, these divisions are really just guides; for example, someone with early-stage dementia might find much joy from the simpler practices. So please feel free to explore the practices within the book fully.

For those seeking a more stimulating practice and who want to try the more challenging practices outlined in Chapter 9, I recommend: a yoga mat (if you do not have one you can start with a towel for seated positions, and a non-slip warm surface, that is, a laminate floor, for other poses); a rectangle yoga block or thick book, for example, a telephone directory; a cushion; a blanket; a yoga strap or normal belt; and a blank wall or pillar.

The practices outlined in Chapters 8 and 11 are mainly chair-based. All these require are a comfortable chair, which can easily be found in most homes or residential care settings. It is important that the person practising can sit up straight, so a cushion might be needed if the seat of the chair slopes backwards. Whether you or the person you are leading is sitting on the floor or on a chair it is important to sit on a block or a cushion and have the hips above the knees. This helps to maintain a natural curve in the spine and enables the front of the body to open fully so the person can take in a full breath. When the knees are positioned above the hips, the upper thighs compress the lower belly, which makes it harder to breathe. This is important in the chair-based sessions, but also very important in the guided relaxations and meditations.

It is also important that the chair is not too high and that the knees are in line with the hips, and that the feet are supported on the floor. It might be useful to have some books or yoga blocks to bring the feet to the right height.

For those living in the late stages of dementia, or those with other health complications, you might prefer the practices shown in Chapter 14. These can be done lying down or sitting on a comfortable chair. For these more relaxed practices you may wish to have a blanket or cushions.

Where to practise

The great thing about yoga is that you can practise anywhere; for example, a normal living room would be fine. However, there are some considerations to bear in mind. Many of those living with dementia might find that they are easily distracted, so I recommend a quiet room where disturbances will be minimised (see below). It is also important to have a well-ventilated room, particularly for the breathing exercises. Having a room with lots of natural light is also beneficial for those practising, although some practices are recommended for the evenings/before bed.

In the summer months, groups I have worked with have really enjoyed practising outside, and there are some specific practices outlined in Chapter 13, such as nature therapy (page 228), that can be done outside.

If practising in a group it is best to arrange the chairs in a circle, with the leader in a position where everyone can see them. I have also had clients in wheelchairs joining in, and in this case, the same considerations about posture mentioned above for chairs applies.

Of course, the more we can do to make our practice space appealing, the more we are likely to practise. Some people like to have a photo of a loved one in their practice space, to remind them that it is not only themself they practise for. Others might like to burn incense or essential oils to help stimulate the senses (and some recommendations for oils to burn can be found on page 211, Chapter 12). Others might prefer to listen to some soft, non-distracting, background music (see below). Popular choices include CDs aimed for reiki or meditation, natural sounds, soft chanting or singing bowls.. It also makes a light sound that can be stimulating and energising for the nervous system. In your practice space you might like to include a picture of an inspiring person, place or symbol. The word 'inspire' comes from the word to 'breathe in' and also 'enthusiasm'. Enthusiastic action helps us to grow our neural connections (see page 84, Chapter 5), so any figure, special object, photo of a special moment, flowers, etc. that help inspire you or the person you are practising with can be used in your practice space.

A note on music: it is best to do yoga in a quiet space so we can focus on the sound of the breath. People living with dementia benefit from periods of silence, and may need extra time to process information given, so having periods of silence in between instructions can be beneficial. However, we all know that homes and care homes have lots of distracting noises, for example, traffic noise, the sounds of other residents or beeping machinery. Therefore, a completely quiet room is often not possible. If it is impossible to soundproof the room, some gentle background music (sometimes known as white noise) can be used to 'mask' unwanted sounds. In my experience I find that instrumental and music with vocal sounds but without words seems to work best. Above I make some suggestions for background music, but this will often depend on a person's personal preference. Feel free to try some of your own favourite soothing sounds.

If you are practising or leading more relaxing sessions I recommend music pulsed at about 60 beats per minute. Slower music has been shown to help people take things in, and has been reported to improve studying performance. However, for the more dynamic sessions, you could try music at about 120 beats per minute. When combined with the right beats, studies have shown that athletes who use music use less oxygen than athletes who do not listen to music.

When to practise

In ancient India it was believed that it was best to practise yoga at dusk or dawn, as these were the most auspicious times of the day. However, with busy modern schedules and personal preferences, it is beneficial to practise yoga at any time of the day (rather than not at all!).

Ideally it is best to practise yoga first thing in the morning before breakfast, when the stomach is empty and the mind is fresh. However, for many living with dementia, this may be impractical, and other times of day might be more appropriate for different sequences. I have provided specific sequences in Chapter 12 that are great for those who wake up raring to go. Another sequence is called restorative poses (see page 73, Chapter 4), which is great for evening time, and will help you or those you are practising with fall asleep. The relaxing yoga for better sleep sessions, including yoga nidra (see page 234, Chapter 14) and restorative poses, can take place after the evening meal or before a nap. If you are practising yourself, try to practise regularly.

A little bit each day is better than an hour one day and then nothing for days. Make yoga your everyday activity, like brushing your teeth.

In many residential care environments finding times to fit in a yoga session may be difficult, and bearing this in mind I have provided activities that can last from 10 minutes to one hour. I have also provided some 'rescue remedies' – short activities that can be used to calm an anxious person, deal with anger or help someone sleep – such as journey of awareness (page 131, Chapter 8), or pushing away the clouds (page 70, Chapter 4).

If running an active group session, practising first thing in the morning may be impractical, and so mid-morning or mid-afternoon is advised. It is best to wait a couple of hours after eating, and not to practise when the residents are too sleepy.

When starting a group session in a residential care environment, it is best to start with small groups of clients who you, or a member of the care staff, think will benefit. This will help build your confidence teaching these yoga sessions or if you are a yoga teacher working with people living with dementia. After you have built your confidence and are familiar with a range of sequences, I recommend teaching those who at first seem less responsive, or those living with more advanced stages of dementia.

In my experience, once yoga sessions start in a residential care environment, word often spreads via the staff or residents, and the yoga practices will spread throughout the home. If you are an activities coordinator, care worker or yoga teacher particularly interested in starting yoga within your home, please see the text box on the next page that provides some tips!

Yoga can be fantastic for care homes. It helps residents with coordination, balance, anger and anxiety issues. It can also be fantastic for staff as it gives them real, developable skills, which benefit those they are caring for and also themselves. My study shows that yoga can improve the overall atmosphere in the whole home.

Important things to remember

The main thing in any practice is that it should be enjoyable, and make those doing it feel good. When we practise ourselves, or with others, it is important to remember that all activities are optional. In many of the sequences I have designed I have provided a variety of options. For example, if someone cannot move an arm or lift a leg, an alternative is given. If you are doing the exercises with others, it is important to always demonstrate the easiest option first, rather than showing the most difficult one. Check who can do the first option, and then, if many can, you can give the slightly harder option. It is important to make sure everyone feels that they are included and can do some of the class. This helps establish camaraderie and group bonding.

It is fine to laugh and smile during the sessions as this really can help to release tension, and this book contains some specific exercises (such as the lion's breath outlined on page 188, Chapter 10), which are bound to raise a smile! These are great for raising the mood of a class, and engaging people if they seem uninterested or disengaged. The sessions should be fun and enjoyable.

If at any point you, or anyone you are doing the classes with, feels fatigued or your breath gets laboured, stop and rest immediately. Take a moment to close your eyes, take some deep breaths, and only start again if you feel well enough.

With any deep breathing, if someone has low blood pressure, they should return to normal breaths if they feel at all faint.

RUNNING YOGA SESSIONS IN A RESIDENTIAL CARE ENVIRONMENT

The research project I ran, called 'Yoga for People Living with Dementia in Residential Care Settings', was supported by Patients First, a innovative fund that supports projects that seek to improve people's lives and their experiences of care. The project team learned skills to help get the best results possible by working collaboratively within the care environment. So, you might ask yourself, what does this mean in practice?

Care workers do a fantastic job! It always surprises me that society often values people who sit in offices moving money around more than those people who care for ourselves, our family members and loved ones. After working hard for many years, perhaps raising a family and contributing to society in so many ways, don't we, ourselves, or those we care for, deserve to have high-level care and compassion as we grow older? Often care workers have great ideas and really want to make a difference to those people they care for; however, they might be limited by staff shortages or being overworked. Care work can be physically and mentally demanding, and often carers suffer from stress. Yoga can be a fantastic initiative to introduce into any caring environment. It is inexpensive to implement and benefits not only those living in the home, but also their carers and other workers. It is fun, keeps staff active, can reduce issues such as back and shoulder pain, and can reduce staff stress levels.

If you are a care worker, having a high level of support for starting yoga sessions in your place of work can be a prime factor in their success, as others within the home will need to help residents attend the sessions. Below I suggest some ways of getting this support within your home.

Discuss the practice with the home manager. You could choose some of the facts or statistics outlined in 'How yoga works' in Chapter 1 to talk to them about. For example, you might want to discuss the effects of yoga on cognitive impairment, depression, anxiety or falls.

You could also show the manager the photos in this book or one of the accompanying videos to demonstrate that the sequences are gentle and appropriate. The videos can be accessed at www.jkp.com/voucher using the code PLAHAYYOGA. Given that many of those living with late-stage dementia might find verbal communication difficult, involving them in yoga sessions can provide a fantastic way of providing meaningful activities.

You might also like to get other staff within your home to try a few of the activities, and I highly recommend activities such as three-part breath on page 61, Chapter 4, neck stretches on page 152, Chapter 8, and the mettā exercise on page 109, Chapter 6 as short, suitable, effective and great to share.

Notes for teachers and session leaders

As with any movement and breath-based practice it is really important for the teacher or session leader to recognise and acknowledge their own energy levels and emotional state before they enter the room. This will affect how the session goes. For example, if the person taking the class is stressed and anxious, this will come across in the way they teach. Therefore, before you begin teaching, take stock of how you are feeling (i.e. tired/energetic, happy/sad, focused/distracted etc.). Acknowledge this energy, and then take a few deep breaths to find yourself as a teacher, and know that for the duration of the practice, you are there for your students.

It is also important to sense the energy levels of the clients and closely observe their reactions to the movements. If you feel the energy level is dipping, it may be possible to pick up the pace a little. If you see the clients are not keeping up, slow down the movements, and you can always introduce a short pause/chance to reconnect with the breath.

As with any physical or breath-based practice, it is really important that the teacher has experienced the movements/breath work themselves. This way we can teach with authenticity. I therefore recommend doing the session a few times before teaching it.

If you are already a yoga teacher this is great, as I am sure there is much experience you can bring. However, I would advise caution as people living with dementia or with cognitive impairment may react differently to your usual students. Make sure you are very clear when you introduce yourself, ask everyone their names, and make eye contact with them. Do not rush. It is best to have a member of care staff sitting in the group to minimise disruption, as you might find in the initial stages that people might need to leave the class before the end. When working in care environments I have had people shouting and swearing in classes and, in this case, it is best to remain calm.

Yoga can help people release stored emotions, and I have often had people crying in class, particularly after deep relaxations. This is an important part of the process of letting go. Living with dementia can be a great opportunity to let go, for example, of old habits, ideas about ourselves, our stories and memories. We might feel that there is a sense of constriction of the self and a loss, but there is also a great opportunity to open up to the new experiences that come with dementia. To work with people at this transition is both a blessing and a privilege.

LEADING OR DOING MEDITATION AND GUIDED RELAXATION PRACTICES

Throughout this book I have included a number of guided meditation and relaxation exercises. These involve scripts that can be read out or recorded. I have included a couple of these as part of the online resources that accompany this book. However, for the others, there are a number of ways to practise the meditations and guided relaxations.

If you are practising yourself, one of the best ways to do these practices is to read the text out aloud whilst recording it, and most modern phones have an easy-to-use record function. When reading, make sure you read slowly and clearly, and allow for lots of pauses, for people to process the information. You can then lie or sit down to listen to the recording. This is helpful, as you will have the recording for future use.

Another great way to practise is to have someone read the text to you while you sit or lie down in a comfortable position with your eyes closed.

Once you have familiarised yourself with the meditations and sequences, you can do them without the instructions as gradually you will remember more and more of the order.

PRINCIPLES AND PRACTICES

There are some key principles to yoga that we should all be aware of, whether we are seasoned practitioners or completely new to yoga. If you are new to yoga, you might find that this section is a bit abstract, but as you move through the sequences and the poses in this book, you may want to refer back to this section, as these are some of the guiding principles of our practice.

Intention

When we do any activity or embark on any project it is useful to set out our intention. This helps us focus our minds and gives people the best experience. This is the same for our yoga practice.

An intention could be a number of things:

- If we have been feeling distracted, our intention could be 'I am focused.'

- If we are tired or not feeling 100 per cent, our intention could be 'I will be soft and gentle on myself.'

- If we are worried about a friend or family member who is ill, our intention could be 'I dedicate this practice to X, may they be happy, well and free from suffering.'

- If we are leading a group in a yoga practice, or are a teacher, our intention could be 'I will guide everyone softly and gently and be aware of their abilities and limitations.'

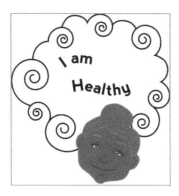

Choose an intention that suits you and/or the group you are working with today.

Breath

How we breathe in yoga is one of its fundamental aspects, and it differentiates true yoga from what I call 'making shapes' yoga. The breath helps to link the outer and inner worlds and our awareness. Therefore, whenever you are practising any yoga, always be aware of your breath. Yoga is well designed, as generally movements that open the chest and expand the natural space of the lungs will occur on an in-breath, and movements that close the lungs will occur on an out-breath. When the breath and movements are combined, it helps us to breathe slowly and more consciously, thereby switching on the positive hormones discussed in Chapter 6.

When we do any breathing exercises, particularly if we are new to them, it is important only to go to the level you are comfortable with. For some people with anxiety, deep breathing and breath holding can make the feelings of anxiousness or claustrophobia worse. While deep breathing can help to lower blood pressure, if someone already has low blood pressure, it can make someone feel faint or dizzy. Therefore, if at any point during any breathing exercises you feel like you are not getting enough breath or you feel anxious, faint or dizzy, always remember to back off. To back off is either to lessen the intensity of what you are doing, or return to your natural and normal breathing pattern. If you are standing, sit or lie down.

Skilful breathing has the ability to help us change our emotional and mental states. Therefore learning to better control the breath is key; however, learning breathing techniques takes time, and it is important not to overdo it when we first start.

Be aware

As well as being aware of our breath, when practising yoga we need to be more aware at all times. So, for example, if you find yourself drifting off during the class and thinking about what you are having for dinner or doing later, bring your attention back to one aspect of the present moment. It could be the sounds around you, the rise and fall of the breath, or any other aspect of the present moment. Awareness is key in yoga, and it is particularly important when it comes to avoiding injury. Specifically be aware of any pain that arises. In yoga we do not say 'no pain, no gain'; we say 'no pain, no pain'. Yoga should never be painful. You might experience sensations as you stretch new parts of your body you are not used to working. However, the way to tell the difference between pain and sensation is often if we are in pain our breath will change and we might not be able to breathe as fully and deeply. If you are ever aware of any pain, always back off and stop the exercise you are doing.

Eye movements

We can tell a lot by our eye movements, and certain eye movement methods have been developed into therapeutic practices. Some researchers have shown that attention and gaze control are affected by specific neurodegenerative disorders, and tracking eye movements can be an early predictor of Alzheimer's and Parkinson's disease. Where we look or gaze in yoga (which is known as our point of drishti) is a very important aspect of yoga. In my classes I have found that when people's eyes wander all around the class, they tend to be less focused and distracted. When someone focuses the eyes in a soft, relaxed way, they are able to relax more fully and be more focused on their inner feelings and world. Fixing the gaze helps to bring our energy inwards; however, it is important to keep the gaze soft. What I mean by a 'soft gaze' is instead of giving something a 'hard' stare, it would be to keep the eyes much softer. For example, hold your hand up in front of you like you are making a thumbs-up sign and stare at your thumb nail like you are giving it the 'hard stare'. Try this for a few minutes, observing your breath. Next, widen your gaze so you are still looking at your thumb, but your peripheral vision is wider. Take a few breaths here, and see if your breath changes in any way. You might be able to notice a slight deepening and lengthening of the breath. This is the gaze we should use in yoga. For more exercises on the gaze, see the eye exercises on page 154, Chapter 8.

Positive attitude

As we have seen, our mind and attitude are governed by the patterns of our thoughts. Therefore, having a positive mental attitude is important. Now I know this might sound difficult, particularly if we are living with dementia or our loved ones have had a recent diagnosis, but trying to remain positive helps us to enjoy the good moments more and remain in the present. Positive thoughts can also help us stay fitter for longer.

Grounding

Grounding is another key principle of yoga. Whatever position we are in, whether it be sitting or standing, we should keep some of our focus on the part of our body that is touching the ground. As we exhale, we should let our weight relax into the ground, and as we inhale, we should feel the body move away from the ground. The more we relax and allow the ground to support us, the more 'connected' and real we can be.

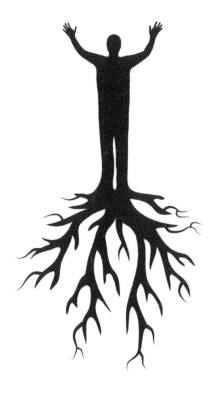

Aligning

Yoga seeks to promote good alignment. Our alignment refers to our body's relationship with itself, for example, the relationship between the hips and the shoulders, or the left side and the right side. Aligning is also about the body's relationship with gravity, which makes balance physically possible. Some exercises to practise alignment are the balance poses such as tree pose (vriksasana) on page 67, Chapter 4 and mountain pose (tadasana) on page 161, Chapter 9.

Yoga contains a mixture of symmetrical and asymmetrical positions, and often in sequences it is common and traditional to practise the right side first and then the left side. However, there is no particular scientific or spiritual reason to start practices on the right side, so although throughout this book I have given instructions for sequences to start on the right side, once you get more familiar with the sequences, practise starting some of these with the left side first. This will help stimulate the brain and avoid doing the sequences by rote.

Modifying

I strongly believe that yoga should be accessible, and that adapted yoga is suitable for all. Modifying a position or sequence means making it suitable for the person doing it. So if, for example, a person can only lift their arms to a certain height in the pose, only instruct them to go this high. If they need to use a chair or a wall to do a pose, this is their modified pose. Yoga is a practice that is constantly changing and adapting, and it is therefore essential to always modify the pose.

Feedback

A key part of modifying involves listening to feedback. There are different types of feedback we can listen to. Feedback from our own bodies can be when we are doing an activity, just after or in terms of how our bodies feel the next day.

If we are working with clients or a family member it is really important to listen to their feedback, including both verbal and physical feedback. As people might be living with late-stage dementia and might not be able to communicate, make a special effort to watch their body language to check they are responding to the activity.

Visualisation

Yogis, coaches and many other health professionals have shown that visualisation of our goals brings many benefits. Visualisation has also been shown to help reduce stress, help us feel happier and can also help us heal better. In Satyananda yoga the teachers recommend that if a student cannot do an exercise, they will benefit greatly from visualising themselves doing it. So, if any poses are not available for you or any of those you are working with at present, try to visualise doing the poses.

CONCLUSION

As we can see from this chapter, there are very few material things we need to progress to the next section of the book. What we do need is an open heart and mind, a willingness to look inside, to be peaceful and still, and also to move consciously and with awareness. The following chapters introduce practical tried and tested techniques and sequences.

CHAPTER 8

SEQUENCES FOR ALL

I have already explained that not much equipment is needed to practise or lead very simple yoga sequences. However, there are some fundamental principles that are needed for all, regardless if you are a teacher, session leader, student, friend or relative. This chapter explores these, and provides some exercises that can be done to develop these skills. One of the great joys of yoga is that the skills developed 'on the mat' or 'in the chair' will be extremely valuable to all those learning them, and can benefit many parts of your life. In this chapter I have simplified my over 20 years' experience of yoga and meditation into simple and easy exercises. If you are new to yoga, please do the exercises yourself first, and observe how you feel before trying them with others.

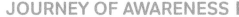

JOURNEY OF AWARENESS

Yoga, mindfulness and meditation are about developing our awareness of the present moment. As daily life becomes more stressful, and perceived demands greater, people become more stressed and distracted. They might regret things they have done in the past, or worry about future events. I am sure we have all had an experience of worrying a lot about something, for example, a meeting with a colleague, or a difficult conversation we need to have, and have been dreading it for days, then finding that when we have the conversation or meeting it was not so bad. After, we berate ourselves and say, 'Why did I spend so much time worrying and getting so stressed? That was stupid.' Or we might worry about seeing a relative who is living with dementia, or a client who is difficult.

Yoga and meditation techniques help us to be in the present moment, and when we are more focused on the present, we can respond to what is happening better, make better decisions and learn to enjoy that moment for what it is. Many people also seek happiness in past memories or perceived future events. And whilst there is absolutely nothing wrong with recalling past happy times, when people dwell too much on their own, or their loved one's past, this can increase their present burden of suffering, especially if they compare their lives now with their previous life. For example, Harvey was a man in his early 80s in the Yoga for Dementia project I worked on. His wife, who was ten years younger, would visit us and often remark to me how Harvey had not always been like he was, and how smart he had been and the life they had had before. Whenever Harvey's wife visited, she would be comparing him with an earlier version of himself, rather than accepting Harvey as he was at the time. This resulted in additional stress and tension, which I suspect Harvey picked up on during her visits. When we work with those living with dementia we have to be aware that they pick up on our moods, if we are angry, stressed or down. The following exercise is key to becoming aware of our moods.

This exercise has its origins in Buddhist practice, but has been adapted and simplified. One of the beauties of this practice is that it can be done by anyone, anywhere. It can be adapted to take more than 20 minutes or only 5.

You can do this with a friend by reading the text below out to each other, or you can read and record the text and then listen to it. Be sure to include lots of pauses and gaps. Once you have familiarised yourself with the text, you can practise yourself by remembering the sequence in your mind, or guide an individual or group through the exercise.

The practice

Find a comfortable seat – this can be on a chair or sitting on the floor crossed-legged, or even lying down. Make sure the body is symmetrical and the spine is straight. Adjust the head so the neck is comfortable. Lick your lips and swallow a couple of times. This helps to relax the jaw.

Now close your eyes. Begin by bringing your awareness to the sounds around you. Start with those that are farthest away first. See if you can move your focus from sound to sound like a bee or a butterfly moving from flower to flower. Just rest the awareness on one sound, and then move to the next sound.

Try to notice if your mind starts to categorise the sounds or judge them. For example, it might be telling you that the sound of machinery or coughing is bad, and the sound of birds is good.

Try to ignore this judging part of the brain, and just focus on moving your awareness from one sound to another.

Next, move your awareness to sounds that are closer. It could be sounds in the building or the room you are in.

Bring your awareness to the sound of your breath. Listen to the sound of the in-breath, the sound of the out-breath and the pauses in between. Do not try to change the breath; simply listen to the sounds.

From the sounds of the breath, bring your attention to the sensations involved in breathing, for example, the feeling of the chest rising and falling, the feeling of the breath in the belly, or maybe the sensation of the cool air entering the nostrils and the slightly warmer air leaving them.

However you notice the feelings and sensations associated with breathing, just focus on that. Once you have focused on the breath for a while, see if you can notice if the breath feels long or short, deep or shallow. Notice if it is even or uneven.

Next, begin to notice other physical sensations within the body. It could be an ache or pain, or the feeling of clothes touching the skin, or the contact of the body on the chair or on the floor. It doesn't matter what you notice; simply notice the physical sensations within the body. As with the sounds you might begin to find that the mind starts judging the sensations or providing a running commentary, for example, 'Oh the chair feels hard, my bum hurts.' Or 'My right shoulder feels really tight, I must remember to wear my bag on the other shoulder.' And so on and so forth. Try to ignore this internal dialogue, and know that all sensations within the body will arise, stay for a while, and pass. Therefore try not to get caught up in them, observe them for a short while, and then move on to the next sensation.

From focusing on the physical sensations move your attention to the emotions within the body. Recognise if you are feeling happy or sad; energetic or lethargic; strong or weak; confident or shy; calm or anxious. Maybe you feel many different emotions or maybe you feel none of the above. This doesn't matter; like the sensations, all emotions will arise, stay for a while, and then pass.

Try to be present with the emotional feelings within the body. If there is a strong emotional feeling, try to notice whereabouts in the body the feeling arises – is it in the heart, the stomach, the brain, the shoulders, etc.?

Next, move your attention to your mind and the space behind the forehead where the thoughts play out. Try to notice if the mind is busy with lots of thoughts coming in, if it is slower, if it is pre-occupied with one particular thought or many. Again, try to avoid judging the mind; just sit or lie down quietly and allow thoughts to come and go. Stay here for some time.

Once you are ready to come out of the exercise, move slowly back through the stages, spending a little time in each. So, from mind awareness to emotional awareness. Then move your attention back to your physical body, then narrow it down to the physical sensations of breathing for a few breaths. Next, take your attention to the sound of the breath. Then finally, to the external sounds.

When you are ready to get up and move, take a few deeper breaths. Slowly open your eyes, stretch and move a bit, and observe how you feel.

Record any particular observations in your notebook.

How it works

This practice, by using various levels of awareness to access the present moment, helps us learn how to come back to the present at any given moment, for example, by just focusing on sounds or our breath. It also helps us recognise the 'judging mind' that compares things, or creates stories or fantasies about our current situation. This part of the mind can learn to dramatise things or react very negatively to situations.

When we learn to step back, observe and sit with our emotions or mental dialogue in a guided meditation exercise, we are much more likely to be able to access this ability in our everyday lives. For example, instead of worrying incessantly about what our future might look like, we can learn to focus on where we are feeling good now. Any situation has positive and negative sides, and I have witnessed first hand the joy that people living with dementia can experience and tap into through the simple practices in this book.

Furthermore, identifying where emotions are felt in the body can help us better understand where we store our emotional energy. For example, if we always feel tense in our shoulders, we might want to pay special attention to these, and do some shoulder exercises. This practice is a form of pratyahara (withdrawal of the senses), which helps us move from the distracted outside world into the inner world.

DHYANA, FOCUSED CONCENTRATION

As we explored in Chapter 3, dhyana, the seventh limb of yoga, comes from the ancient Indian language Sanskrit word dhyai, which means 'to think of'. Dhyana involves focused concentration and meditation on a point of focus with the intention of knowing it. This can help lead us to the ultimate goals of yoga. Below I have described an exercise that can be done with a partner or alone, and can be used to develop this skill.

Eye-gazing meditation or trataka is an emotional cleansing tool that helps people to connect and feel compassion for each other. It also increases the ability to be present for someone else. It can be done with a family member, a person living with dementia, someone you work with, or alone with a mirror. You might initially feel awkward about doing this practice with someone else, but please be open-minded and give it a try.

The practice

Sit facing each other in chairs. If you are sitting, you can put a pillow on your lap and hold hands if you like. Try to ensure you are sitting close enough that you do not have to lean forwards. Gaze into your partner's eyes, keeping the gaze soft and relaxed by defocusing them slightly. Try to relax and breathe slowly through your nostrils. The objective of the meditation is about how you experience your partner, finding out more about them without words. Be open to this experience. Observe your partner's face, their eyes, their expressions. As you gaze you might feel a range of emotions such as tension, anger, sadness, awkwardness etc. Try to stay with the feelings; just be there. Don't worry – nothing is going to happen from just sitting, apart from that you might learn something. If you haven't got a partner to practise with, try practising by gazing into your own eyes in a mirror.

After you have finished the practice, take a few minutes to record your observations in your notebook.

How it works

This practice is great for people with all stages of dementia. Often people living with more advanced dementia might find being asked questions and not having the skills to respond very stressful. I have also noticed from my own experience that visits to someone living with dementia can be made up of an over-bright and cheery monologue from the person visiting. When doing trataka or eye gazing with someone, we are not asking them for anything; we are simply observing them and being there for them without any expectations or judgements. We will find as we relax into this practice our breath will often deepen and we will feel more comfortable with the person. This can be wonderful for later interactions with them, and helps create bonding and connection.

PRANAYAMA, OR BREATH AWARENESS IN THE SPINE

This introductory exercise helps us develop awareness of the upward and downward-moving energy in the body. In general the in-breath brings with it an upward-moving energy known as prana, and the outbreath a downward-moving energy known as apana. The ability to feel this breath will help with many of the physical and breathing exercises within this book.

To do this exercise, sit comfortably in a chair and again, either ask someone to read you the instructions below, or you could record them.

The practice

Yoga is a practice of awareness and attention, so next we bring the focus to the body. Close your eyes now.[1] First, sense your feet on the floor or mat. Spread your toes and feel the heaviness of the feet and legs. Push your feet down into the earth. Then allow the whole awareness to go into your legs, and note any sensations in your legs and hips.

---

1   Often with elderly clients they might feel anxious (especially if they are new to yoga), and might not wish to close their eyes. If this is the case, it is helpful to remind them that they are in a safe environment and nothing will happen once their eyes are closed; there is nothing to see, and they are not going to miss anything. It is also worth reminding them that closing their eyes helps them to sense inwards and reconnect with the breath.

Then move your awareness to the upper body. Feel the breath moving into your belly. Take some nice, long, deep belly breaths… and then allow the breath to move into the upper chest and into the lungs. Really focus on the rise and fall of the chest as you breathe. Feel the breath move into the sides of the body, and imagine the ribs fanning out like an accordion on each in-breath. Feel the heart lifting a bit higher towards the sky as you inhale. As you exhale, feel the shoulder blades dropping down the back, easing any tension away.

On your next inhale feel the crown of the head lifting higher, then exhale and allow your arms and hands to be heavy. Next, feel the breath moving into the spine. As you inhale feel the breath travelling up the spine, starting from the base of the body moving up, vertebrae by vertebrae. As you exhale see if you can drop the shoulders a bit further down the back, and allow yourself to feel a bit heavier and a bit more relaxed. As you exhale see if you can feel that the exhale is going down into the floor, connecting you with the earth.

With each inhalation feel a bit taller, and feel the spine extend and grow towards the sky, like a flower moving towards the sun. With each exhalation try to feel as though you have arrived a little more into the body and feel the connection, like your feet are growing roots that extend into the floor and earth below you.

Pause and breathe for a while, observing these sensations.

To come out, take all your attention down to your arms, and feel your hands resting against your legs. Now take your full attention to the palms of your hands, and feel all the sensations in your hands – the feeling of air against the skin, the feeling of the clothes you are wearing.

Next, slowly (without opening your eyes) lift your hands out in front of you – make this movement really slow and sense the hands moving through the air. Repeat this movement a few times, lifting the arms on the inhale and lowering them on the exhale. Eventually bring the hands to touch at the heart centre, feeling the tips of the fingers and palms touching.

We will come back to some more detailed exercises later in the book. However, now I introduce two chair-based sequences that are suitable for all. They are a great introduction to yoga, and will help those new to leading yoga-based sessions as well as those wishing to practise by themselves at home. They help to tone and strengthen the whole body in a safe and sustainable way.

  ## SEQUENCE 1: RISE AND SHINE!

This short, dynamic session is good for raising energy levels and is best practised either first thing in the morning or just before lunch. It is a great introductory session for those who are new to yoga. The whole sequence can take about 30–45 minutes. However, feel free to modify it or shorten sections of the sequence when you first start practising yourself or with others. Ideally you, or those you are practising with, will have shoes off and be in loose socks.

Grounding into the feet

a) Settle into the chair, move your weight from side to side in order to find the left and right sides of your buttocks. Then, sitting up straight, take some deep breaths up and down the spine (see 'Pranayama, or breath awareness in the spine' on page 136).

b) Find your feet on the footrest or floor by spreading and pressing the feet into the floor (make sure the knees are in line with the hips – see 'Before you begin' on page 117, Chapter 7).

c) Wiggle your toes, and find the balls of the feet and heels by rocking the feet forwards and backwards, and then press down into the floor, activating the legs.

d) Lift all ten toes, and keeping them raised, lift and lower the big toe (five times). Then lift and lower the little toe (five times).

e) Wiggle all ten toes again, then spread the toes and lower them to the ground.

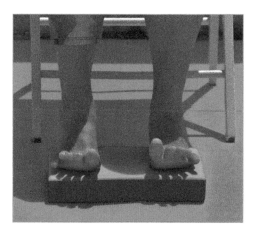 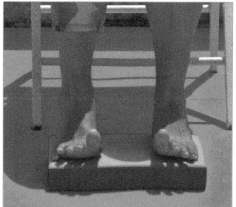

Grounding into the feet helps activate the legs and produces strength and stability through the feet and legs, thereby improving balance. Focusing on the feet also gets people's attention away from the thoughts in their heads. The feet have a great capacity for becoming more dexterous and responsive, and are full of acupressure and reflexology points.

If you or someone you are practising with does not have great control of their toes, just encourage them to try their best or just wiggle their toes. Any movements in the feet will be activating nerves and muscles and are therefore beneficial.

Lengthening the spine

a) Exhale, pressing down into the feet.

b) Inhale, and feel the spine lift and lengthen from the feet up.

c) Use your hands to press down into the sides of the chair to extend the spine further to the ceiling.

Leg exercises

a) Lift your right leg off the floor so it is in line with your knee. If the foot cannot get up this far, don't worry; the main thing is that it is off the floor. If you need to, support your torso by holding on to the sides of the chair. Next, exhale and point your toe away. Then inhale and flex (draw the toes towards you) and lower (repeat three times).

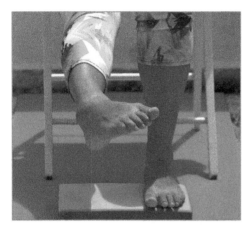 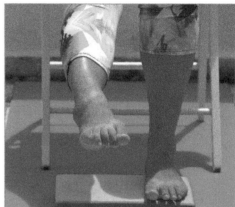

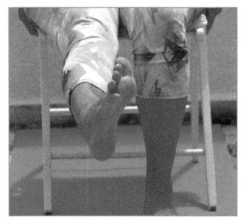

b) With the leg raised make small circles with the foot and toes first one way and then the other, increasing the diameter of the circle each time (repeat three times each side).

c) Then invert and exert the foot by bringing the inside edge (big toe side) of the foot towards the inner ankle, and then the outside edge (little toe side) of the foot towards the outside ankle (repeat three times).

d) Repeat (a)–(c) on the left-hand side.

e) Next, bring the feet back to the floor. On an inhale breath, squeeze your thighs together (imagine squeezing a sponge in between the knees). At the same time, lift your pelvic floor. Exhale to relax. Repeat this five times, seeing if you can hold the squeeze and lift a little longer each time.

f) Tap the legs together, and lift and lower the legs to knee-high (still tapping) (three times). If difficult to do both legs together, simply lift and lower one leg at a time.

g) To finish, pat down the legs with your hands from top to bottom. First pat down the fronts, then the inner side of the legs, and then the outer sides. This part of the sequence helps to strengthen and activate the legs. The pelvic floor is one of our key postural muscles, and this exercise is good for bladder control.

Twists

Twists help to detox by increasing the flow of blood to the muscles and organs, and can improve back health. They also help to refresh the neural pathways.

a) Inhale and reach the arms up in line with the shoulders, and then exhale, twist to the right, bringing the hands on to the arms of the chair, then inhale, reach up and repeat to the left-hand side.

b) Repeat two times, and on the final side, lift the leg up on the same side you are twisting to, and then remain in position for three to five breaths.

c) Focus on squeezing the pelvic floor and lifting on the inhalations, and as you exhale, squeeze in the belly and twist a little further. You can turn your head in the same direction of the twist, or in case of any neck issues, keep your head central and in line with the spine.

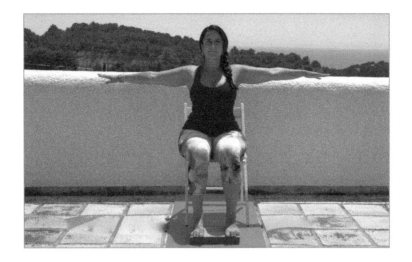

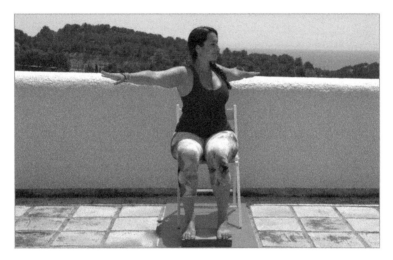

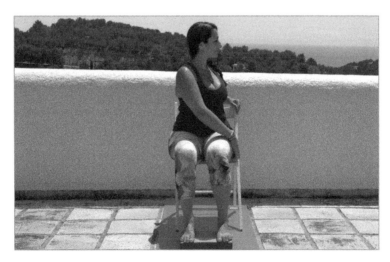

Seated sun salutations, and cat and cow through the spine

Seated sun salutations help to mobilise the spine.

a) Inhale, lift your hands high above the shoulders, palms facing forwards and stretch the spine tall.

b) Exhale, bow down towards the floor, resting your hands on your thighs or shins.

c) Inhale, straighten your spine and look up, resting your hands on your knees or shins and keeping the torso close to the legs.

d) Exhale, and bow the head again towards the knees.

e) Inhale, lift the head and torso back to the start position.

f) Repeat three times.

g) On the last time rest the head forward, shaking out the head and neck.

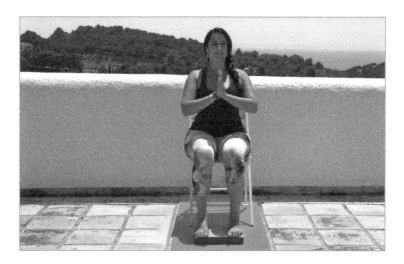

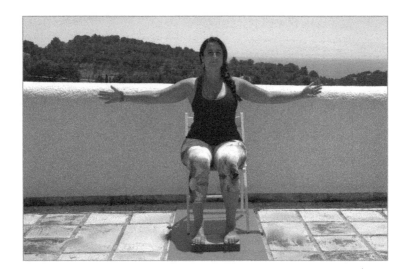

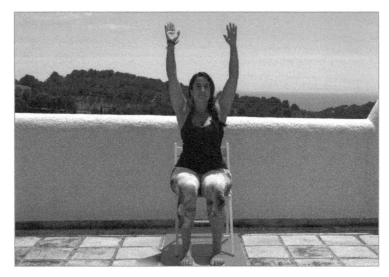

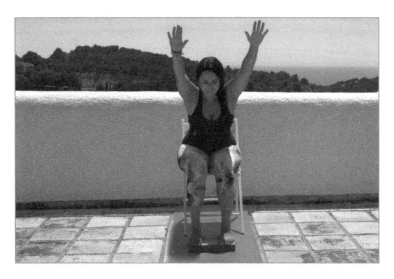

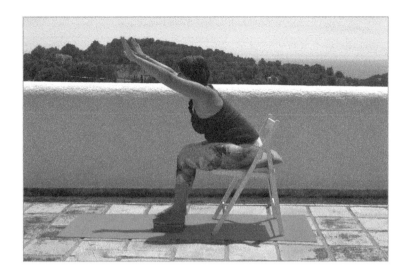

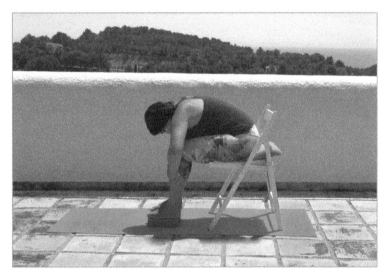

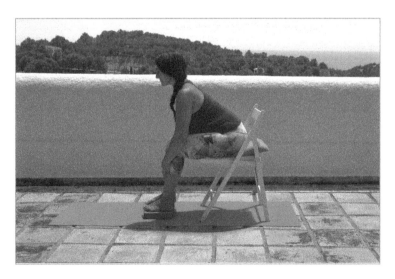

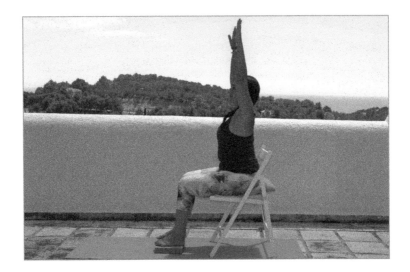

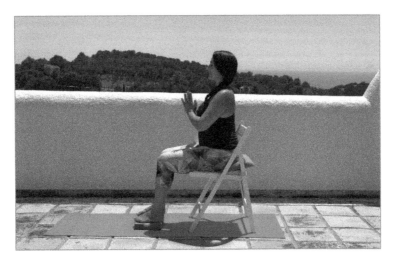

Swimming/running/cycling

The next part of the sequence can be quite aerobic, and can be made more or less energetic depending on how you or the people you are leading are feeling. It helps raise energy levels and gets the blood flow running. These movements mimic natural movements of the body. As you are going through the sequence imagine you are swimming, running or cycling in a nice environment. Sometimes it helps to raise energy levels and keep the sessions interesting to encourage people to imagine they are running for a bus, and getting them to go a little bit faster and faster. At the end you can say 'Ah, caught it!' and rest for a bit. You can also use your imagination with the swimming and cycling parts. Sometimes I joke that we are doing a triathlon in this section!

It is important to include lots of rests and really observe how people are doing.

a) Make swimming motions with the arms. First breast stroke, then back stroke, and then front crawl.

b) With the feet make small running movements, then progress to using the arms as well (if this is not too much effort for you or those you are working with).

c) Holding the arms of the chair, make cycling motions with your legs.

  ### Breathing into the heart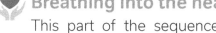

This part of the sequence focuses on lengthening the front of the body. It is a great counter-pose to age-related hunching of the back.

a) Take your hands behind the back, with the palms facing down on the floor; turn your fingers backwards.

b) Use your arms to lift the spine and take the heart towards the ceiling, leaning back slightly if this is comfortable.

c) Breathe directly into the heart space, taking five to ten breaths. Imagine you are breathing into your heart and nourishing and nurturing your heart with these practices.

Shoulder-opening sequence

This part of the sequence is great as it focuses on moving with the breath. It is also great for carers, as it helps to take the shoulders through a full range of movements and really helps release shoulder tension. You can view this part of the sequence on the online resources accompanying this book (available at www.jkp.com/voucher using the code PLAHAYYOGA).

a) Take your hands to your heart in a prayer pose.

b) Inhale, lift your hands above your head (palms facing forwards), stretch your hands as high as is comfortable.

c) Exhale, turn your thumbs out so your palms face up and take your hands down (in line with the chest).

d) Inhale (imagine holding a tray) and draw your hands back so they come in line with the rib cage, lifting your heart up and forwards.

e) Exhale, take your hands back to your heart in a prayer pose.

f) Inhale, take your arms out wide to either side and in line with the chest.

g) Exhale, twist to the right, taking your left hand to your heart, looking to the right thumb.

h) Inhale, back to centre.

i) Exhale, twist to the left, taking your right hand to your heart.

j) Inhale, back to centre.

k) Exhale, bow your head and fold forwards.

l) Inhale, back to the start.

Repeat three to five times.

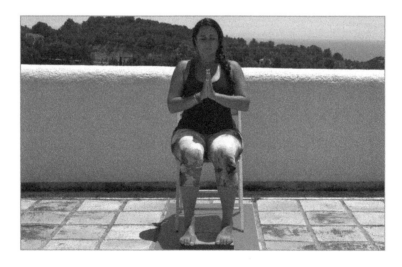

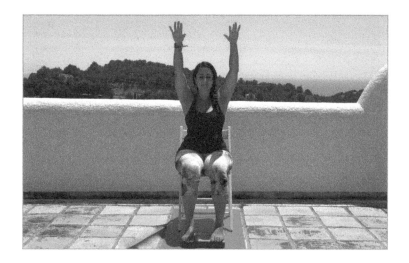

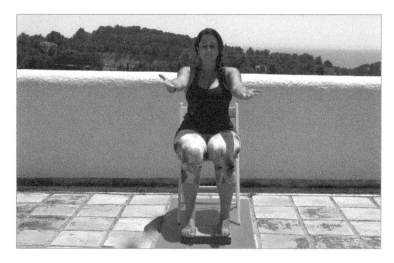

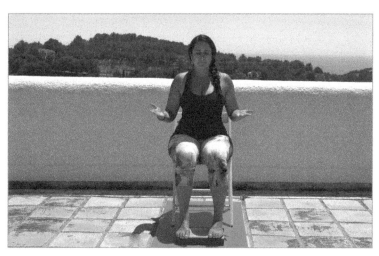

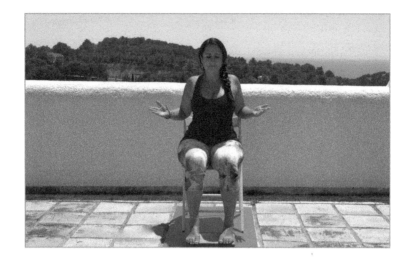

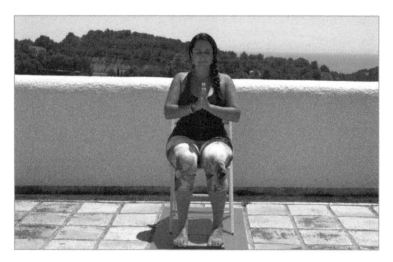

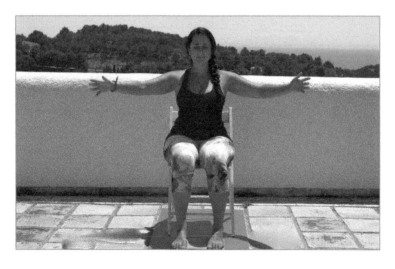

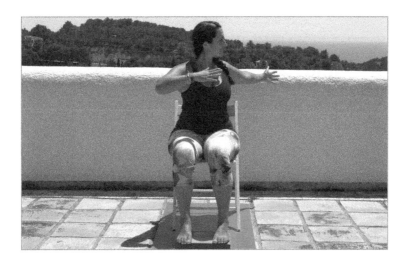

Finishing

You can finish this sequence with the journey of awareness (see page 131). Later on in the book we learn other guided meditation and relaxation practices; however, it is best to focus on familiarising yourself with one or two practices to start with. Once you and/or the people you are working with are comfortable with guided relaxation, you can then use different guided relaxations to finish the sequences.

SEQUENCE 2: FEELING GOOD FROM TOP TO TOE!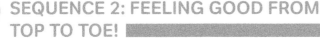

This simple and effective general chair-based lesson is good for a large majority of those living with dementia. It is best if you have some mobility and those you are working with are able to follow instructions. It is a top to toe sequence, and is also good for cancer, anxiety, depression and insomnia.

Settling in and arriving in the body

This practice helps us to calm our minds, and switch on our internal state of awareness.

    a) Settle into the chair (see page 138, Sequence 1, Grounding into feet).

b) Do the journey of awareness exercise (see page 131).

c) Feel the breath in the spine (see 'Lengthening the spine' on page 139).

Neck circles

This exercise warms up and gently stretches the muscles of the neck. However, be sure only to move to your ability; do not over-stretch or strain your neck.

a) Imagine a pencil on the tip of your nose.

b) Begin to make small circles in a clockwise direction, imagining you are drawing a small circle on the wall opposite. Gradually start to spiral out these circles, making them bigger and bigger. Focus on the feelings in the neck and the muscles gently moving and stretching.

c) Once you have reached your maximum capacity, begin to spiral back into the centre.

d) Repeat in a counter-clockwise direction.

Neck stretches

The neck is a key part of the body as it is where all the nerves travel up to the brain and hence lots of messages are transmitted through it. In nursing homes lack of movement often causes a tightening and restriction of the neck. Please be mindful if someone has any neck injuries or has had a tracheostomy.

a) Inhale, lift your head to look at the ceiling, and exhale, lowering your head to look down to the floor. Move slowly with the breath, and go a bit further each time (being careful not to bend the back). Repeat three times.

b) Next, turn your head from right to left, slowly. Exhale to turn the head, and inhale to move the head back to the centre. Try to imagine that you are oiling your neck with your breath.

c) Then take your right ear to your right shoulder. Lift your right hand over your left ear to encourage a gentle opening. In this movement avoid pulling with the hand – it is more about using weight and gravity to assist the stretch.

    d) Turn your head to face down to look at the right thigh. This should move the stretch around to the back of the neck.

Repeat (a)–(d) on the left-hand side.

    e) Next, interlace your fingers and take both hands behind the neck. With the base of the thumbs, lift the bottom ridge of the skull towards the ceiling. You should feel a nice stretch in the back of the spine.

    f) Keeping the back straight, take the chin to the chest with the elbows either side of the ears.

    g) Finish by gently self-massaging the back of the neck, face and jaw with your hands and fingers. You can use your fingertips to gently smooth over the forehead and circle the temples. Pay particular attention to where the upper and lower jaw meet, as lots of tension is stored here. You can also yawn and stretch your face.

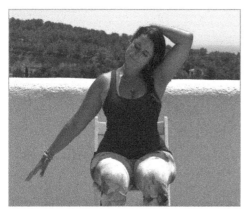
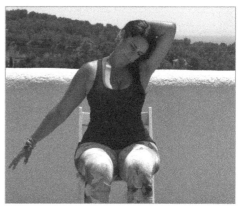
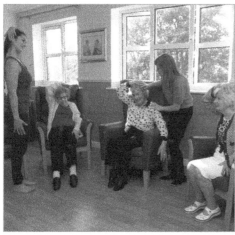
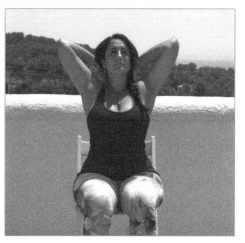

Eye exercises

If needed, please rest your arms in between the different parts of this sequence. These eye exercises help to relax the eyes and create moisture, and are especially good for dry eyes. They also help to stretch and work the eye muscles (which can get weak from focusing in one place, for example, if you or those you are working with watch a lot of TV). Coordinated subtle movements also help to develop neurological pathways.

a) Palming: rub your hands to create warmth and then cover your eyes with your palms. This should create darkness behind the palms. Next, blink your eyes a few times and open them into darkness. Imagine you are breathing in the darkness through your eyes. Repeat this three times.

b) Hold your right arm straight in front of you, and lift your index finger like you are pointing it. Gaze at your fingertip and make large circles with the arm and finger, moving it up, out to the side, down and around to the start position. Repeat this three times, following your finger with your eyes.

c) Then bring your finger to the tip of your nose, and then away from you slowly and then back again. Try to keep the focus on your fingernail at all times. Repeat this three times.

Repeat (b)–(c) with the left finger.

d) Next, slowly look up and down five times, then left and right five times, then diagonally from one side to another five times. Try not to move your head; just focus on moving your eyes.

e) Once you have practised moving the eyes slowly, as in (d), you can then move the eyes rapidly, building up gradually to about ten times.

f) To finish, blink a few times and repeat the palming exercise (a) above.

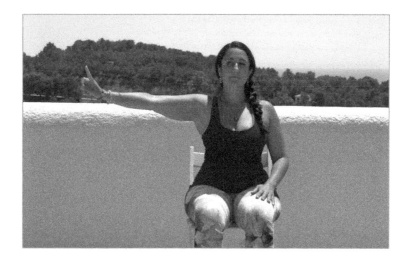

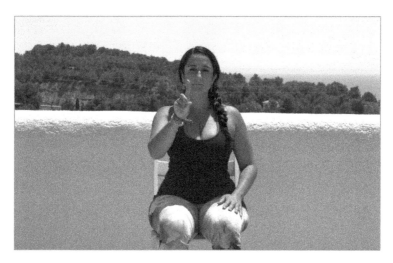

The following exercises help to open the chest and the front of the body. They also help to open the spine. If the chest is tight, the cat and cow movements can be quite small.

Shoulders

a) Begin by rolling your shoulders forwards and backwards a few times.

b) Next, bring your fingertips on to the shoulders with your elbows out to the side. Then bring the elbows together in front of the chest and make big circles forwards with the elbows.

c) Circle the elbows backwards.

d) Circle the elbows in the opposite direction.

e) Finish by opening and closing the spine in a cat and cow motion (see page 72, Chapter 4).

Dynamic rainbow side stretches and twists

These movements help to lengthen the side body and increase lung capacity. The twist helps to detox by increasing the flow of blood to the muscles and organs, can improve back health, and can also stimulate the digestive organs.

a) Reach up to the ceiling with both arms. Then, whilst wiggling the fingers, sway the arms and torso to the left and right (a bit like you are painting a rainbow in the sky).

b) Repeat three times. On the last time take the right hand to the arm of the chair and stretch the left hand up and over – palm facing down and focusing on taking three big breaths into the side ribs. Repeat to the left hand side.

c) Twists to left and right: reach the arms up high and then twist to the right; bring the hands on to the arms of the chair, then reach up and repeat to the left side. Repeat two times and on the final side, stay in the position for three to five breaths. Focus on lifting during the inhalations and twisting on the exhalations.

 ## Arms, hands, fingers and wrists

The giving and receiving mudra is good to retain mobility through the hands. The finger and arm movements help to keep strength in the fingers, hands and wrists. They also help with coordination.

a) Giving and receiving mudra: bring your palms together at your heart centre, then, as you exhale, turn the hands forwards, keeping the thumbs together, then bring the backs of the hands together. Keep the wrists together if possible, and complete a full circle of the hands. Practise this way; a few times, then try circling the hands the other way, for example, from the prayer pose turn the palms towards you, the fingers point to the chest and then down. These two mudras make up a moving, giving and receiving mudra, and you can play with alternating them. During this practice it is useful to focus on what you give and receive in life.

b) Lift one hand up in line with your shoulder.

c) Circle the wrist one way and then the other.

d) Lift and lower the arm, pointing the fingers down as the hand rises, and the fingers up as the hand lowers.

e) Stretch out the fingers and then open and close the fingers one at a time (repeat three times), then shake out the hand and relax it down on the knee.

Repeat on the left-hand side.

Seated sun salutations
See the instructions on page 143.

Leg exercises
See the instructions on page 139.

Top to toe relaxation

This is a great simple relaxation method that anyone can learn. It can be practised as part of a sequence, or it can be a great way to unwind after a stressful day. As part of this sequence we do the exercise in a chair, but it can be performed lying down in the corpse pose (shavasana) (see page 76, Chapter 4).

First start with the feet. Breathe in and squeeze the toes and the feet together tightly and clench the muscles in the feet and toes; as you exhale, relax your feet and toes whilst at the same time saying mentally, 'My feet and toes are relaxed.'

Next, move up to your shins and calves and inhale, squeeze and clench the muscles, then exhale, saying 'My shins and calves are relaxed.'

Next, move up the body, sequentially moving on to the thighs, buttocks, belly, chest, shoulders, upper arms, forearms and hands.

Finish with the face by squeezing and clenching the muscles on the face together. Squeeze and tighten the whole body then afterwards relax by saying the words, 'My whole body is relaxed.'

Repeat the final part of the exercise three times, and then take some time to relax completely and observe how you feel.

Once you have practised these classes and the exercises mentioned above a few times, you should hopefully begin to notice their impact on you or those you are practising with. You might like to record your observations in your notebook. This will also help you remember what you have done. If you are feeling more comfortable with the types of movements, you should be ready to explore other sequences in this book. You might be confident to try some standing movements, or feel that more guided meditations and relaxation techniques are appropriate for you and those you are working with.

CONCLUSION

In this chapter we have explored some sequences for all. Together we have learnt a very simple journey of awareness sequence, which we can use as a stand-alone meditation, or before or after other practices. It is a great way of checking in with ourselves and moving from the external to the internal world. I introduce two dynamic sequences, which help exercise our whole bodies: the first is a great morning routine, and the second helps us work our bodies from top to toe! In this chapter we practice focusing our attention by doing some eye exercises, and learn the practice of eye gazing which is a great way of connecting with others. The chapter concludes with a fantastic top to toe relaxation which is a great way of those living with dementia, and their carers to relax and de-stress at any time.

CHAPTER 9

CHALLENGING AND STIMULATING SEQUENCES FOR THOSE WITH EARLY DIAGNOSIS OR MILD COGNITIVE IMPAIRMENT

The sequences and exercises within this chapter are for people with an early diagnosis of dementia: they are for those who are active, and would like to do more challenging yoga poses and activities. They contain a mixture of physical poses and concentration exercises, and are designed to stimulate the body and mind.

Most of the poses and exercises can be done alone, but some are lovely to do with a relative or friend. These sequences and poses are inspired by a number of types of yoga including kundalini and classic hatha yoga (for more information about the different types of yoga, see Chapter 2).

  ## SINGING PRACTICE, KIRTAN KRIYA

The first exercise we will practise is one that has been tried and tested by a team at UCLA (Eyre et al. 2016) who found this had positive impacts on preventing mental decline. This exercise is from the kundalini yoga tradition and is called kirtan kriya. The word kirtan means 'narrating or reciting' of an idea or story, and is often used to describe the singing of devotional music. The word kriya means a set of practices that are used to work towards a certain outcome. So in essence this is a set sequence of practices based on sound. Now while many people may

feel shy about singing or making sounds, sound can be a fantastic way to release tension, focus and stimulate under-used parts of the brain. In fact, music therapy has been successful for those living with dementia (Särkämö et al. 2014). This exercise enables anyone to access the benefits of making sounds.

This singing exercise can be used by anyone who is interested in improving memory loss and brain function. It involves singing or whispering the following sounds 'sa', 'ta', 'na', 'ma'. The sounds represent the cycle of life, with sa representing birth (or infinity), ta representing life, na signifying death, and ma signifying rebirth.

The reciting of the words is combined with a mudra (or hand gesture). Mudras are said to work by changing the subtle balance of energy within the body. In this exercise the thumbs touch the index fingers of each hand on sa, on ta the thumbs touch the middle fingers, on na they touch the ring fingers and on ma they touch the little fingers. Both hands perform the same movements at the same time, which also helps with coordination. Spend a few moments practising making the sounds and touching the fingers to see how simple this exercise is.

In addition to making the sounds, the exercise also involves visualisation (see Chapter 7 for more about the benefits of visualisation). As you chant each sound, imagine that the sound is coming in through the crown of the head and then making a lying down 'L' shape by coming out of the space between the eyebrow centre (sometimes known as the 'third eye point').

Use a clock or timer to softly chime on every second minute, in order to time the exercise.

Now sit in a comfortable position with your spine straight. You can sit on a chair or on the floor in a cross-legged position – whatever is most comfortable for you.

For 2 minutes sing at a normal level the sa, ta, na, ma, whilst at the same time moving the thumb along the tips of the four fingers and visualising the sound moving from the top of the head and in an 'L' shape out through the third eye point each time you make the sounds. You can sing the words quite loudly.

For the next 2 minutes say the sounds in a whisper, again, with the mudras and visualisation.

For the next 4 minutes, say the sounds silently to yourself, with the mudras and visualisation.

Next whisper the sounds for 2 minutes and then for the final 2 minutes sing them out loud. To finish the exercise, inhale deeply, lift your hands above your head, and then bring them down slowly in a sweeping motion as you exhale. Sit still for a while and take a moment to observe how you feel. Write down any observations in your notebook.

SUN SALUTATION, SURYA NAMASKAR

The next series of exercises involve learning a simple sequence of poses that flow into one another. This is an adapted version of a classic sun salutation (surya namaskar). The term 'sun salutation' simply means to welcome the sun. In ancient India it was believed there were many gods, including gods based on the natural elements such as the god of wind and the sun god (surya). Welcoming the sun is one of the most basic and primal forms of expressing gratitude, as the sun on a chemical level supports all life on earth, including our own. In more modern therapeutic approaches light therapy has been shown to be effective for those living with dementia, and exposure to bright light has helped those living with dementia sleep longer and deeper (Hanford and Figueiro 2013). An additional benefit has been a reduction in cognitive decline and symptoms of depression. Therefore, if you want to increase the benefits of doing the sun salutations, you can do them outside, or in a well-lit room.

There are many different versions of sun salutations, ranging from more difficult to easier versions. This simple adapted version is great for beginners. It can also help to stimulate and balance the right and left side of the brain, as it works both sides equally. Coordinating movement and breath helps to stimulate the mind as well as the body.

TADASANA OR MOUNTAIN POSE

Stand in mountain pose (tadasana). This is a very simple but effective standing pose that engages all the muscles and helps us get a sense of the upward-moving and downward-moving energy (known as prana and apana in yoga).

Position your feet so that they point forwards and are under your hips. If you look down and bend your knees you should be able to see the second and third toes disappear behind your knees as you bend them. This ensures your feet and knees are in correct alignment.

Check in with your hips by tilting them forwards and backwards a few times. When they are correctly positioned you should be able to feel length in the lower back and a slight tone in the belly.

Next, take your weight forwards and backwards and gently from side to side, and focus on the different parts of the feet connecting with the floor. After a few breaths come to the centre and feel like you are standing up nice and tall and there is a straight line, from the crown of your head to your feet. Roll your shoulders up towards your ears and then back and down. Adjust the head and neck by moving it slightly from side to side and up and down to ensure that the head is straight and the crown of the head is extending up to the sky or the ceiling. Reach your fingertips down towards the floor to feel a stretch through the arms.

Correct engagement

It is very important when we practise yoga that we ensure the right level of engagement and relaxation, and we will now do an exercise to practise this. Stand in the mountain pose (see page 161) and relax the whole body, feel the heaviness of the body and how the body moves towards the floor; try to notice that the body feels heavy. Next, engage and stretch the whole body until it is tense. Notice what happens to the flow of breath.

Try to relax the body, but not too much that it is in a disengaged state. When we are in this middle state we are like a finely tuned instrument – we are relaxed enough to feel the breath moving through us but not too relaxed that we are not using any energy. This is the correct state of engagement. When we are in this state we feel focused, our attention is in our body, and we are engaged in the activity.

Any activity can be done in a state of awareness and focus, or a state of distraction, or a tense state. The relaxed state of awareness and focus is in itself yoga. So whenever you are doing any exercise within this book, be vigilant and check you are doing it with the awareness and relaxed focus necessary. When we do mountain pose (tadasana) correctly, we should feel like the bottom half of our body is connected and rooting into the floor like the base of a big mountain, and the top of the body and the spine are extending towards the sky and moving freely. As we breathe in we should feel that the energy is moving up the body from the earth, and as we breathe out we should feel like the energy is moving back into the earth. See if you can imagine that you are plugged in and this energy is recharging you.

To move from mountain pose (tadasana) to the sun salutation we must first 'catch the breath'. Catching the Breath is a bit like the way surfers catch a wave or a kite catches the wind. We want to time our movements with the natural pattern or wave (rise and fall) of the breath. To help us find the breath, start by bringing the hands together in anjali mudra, or prayer pose. This mudra (or hand gesture) is a traditional gesture of greeting, and we can use it in this sequence to celebrate the light of the sun in our own hearts. Press the fingers together, lift the heart and the chest, and gaze softly down at the hands. Close the eyes and take a moment to visualise a glowing sun at the centre of your heart.

Next, catch the inhale – sweep the hands down and then out to each side of your body in two wide circles to meet together again above your head. Bring the hands together and down the central line of your body. As the hands sweep up look up and then follow the thumbs down the centre with your eyes. Repeat this movement three or more times, moving the hands up on your inhale and down on the exhale. You can do this as many times as you like until you feel that you are in time with the breath and you have caught the wave of your breath.

Once you are ready to move on, after you have extended your hands overhead and they are touching, exhale, and sweep them out to the side, whilst at the same time bending forwards at the hips to bring your hands on to your thighs or shins. Keep your hands on the shins, bend the knees slightly and inhale as you look forwards, extending the spine. Exhale and take the forehead towards the legs. Bend the knees, push into the feet, then inhale to come all the way back to standing again, sweeping the hands out to the side, overhead and back to prayer pose (anjali mudra). Again, repeat this movement until you feel like you have got the hang of it, and are moving with the breath.

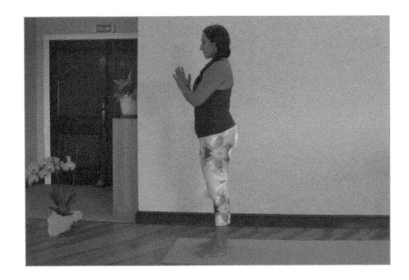

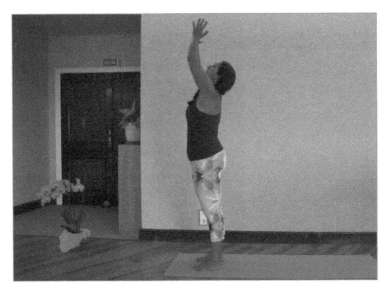

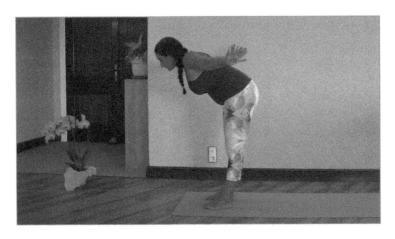

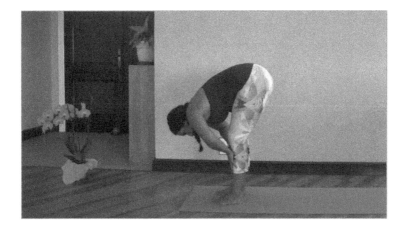

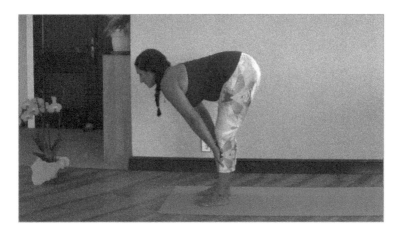

Once you feel comfortable with this movement and your spine feels a bit warmer you can progress to the next step. After you next fold forwards, bend the knees to take the hands either side of the feet. Step your right foot backwards to come into a pose called low lunge. Low lunge involves having the back knee and foot on the floor and the front knee bent. It is important that the front knee is above the front ankle so the shin is in a straight line.

Stabilise the feet by pushing down into them, then inhale and lift the torso, sweeping the hands out to the side and above the head to meet in prayer pose (anjali mudra). Exhale and sweep the arms back and out to the side as you bend forwards, to take the hands either side of the front foot. Step back so both knees are on the floor in a kneeling plank.

Kneeling plank

To do kneeling plank have both knees on the floor and your shoulders over your wrists. Your body should make a straight line from your shoulders to the back of the knees. Next, exhale and lower the whole body to the floor, so you will be lying face down on the floor.

Place your hands either side of your chest, palms facing down, and press your hips and legs down into the floor. Inhale and lift your chest and head. Exhale and move your head back and down. Move your hands forwards slightly, exhale and take your bottom back towards your heels and stretch your hands out in front of you into a pose called child's pose (balasana).

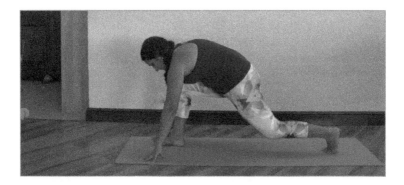

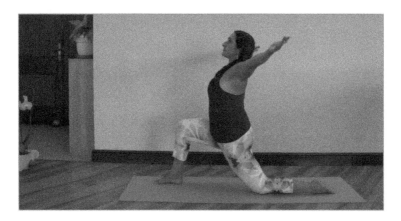

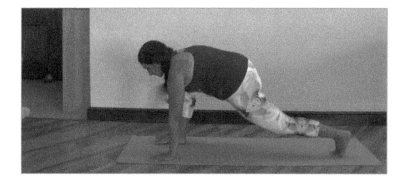

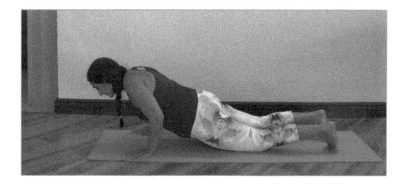

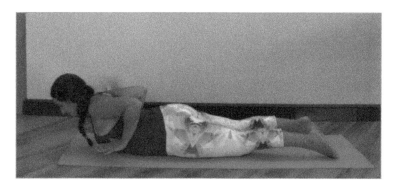

Child's Pose, Balsana

Child's pose is a wonderfully nurturing pose and can be lovely when we feel like we want to move inside and retreat into our shells. To do this pose correctly, bring your big toes together and have your knees wide, then extend your tailbone down towards your bottom. Have your chest and head close to or on the ground, and your hands can either be extended out in front of you, palms to the ground, or resting either side of your hips, with palms facing up to the sky. Rest for a while in the pose and try to remember the steps you have taken to get here.

Downward-facing dog

When you are ready to move on, extend your hands once again on to the floor in front of you. Press them down, tuck your toes underneath your feet and then push your bottom up to the ceiling, so you stretch your body equally through the legs, torso and arms. The knees can remain bent, but it is key to turn your hips up to stretch the back fully. This pose is called downward-facing dog (adho mukha svanasana). Stay in this pose for a while if it feels comfortable.

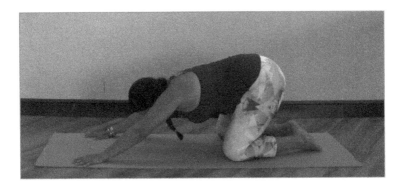

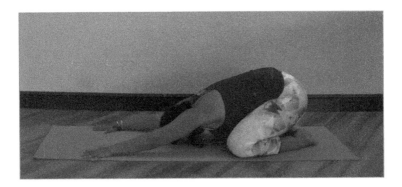

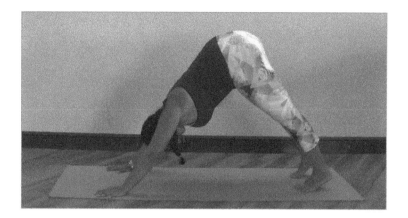

When you are ready to move to the next pose, lift your right leg behind you and exhale, sweep it forwards and step it in between your hands. It might take a few steps to get there. Drop your back knee to arrive once again into a low lunge. Inhale, sweep your hands out to the sides to touch at the top, exhale, and move your hands down to either side of your front foot. Then tuck your back toes under and step forward into a forwards fold.

Inhale, look forwards extending the spine, exhale and return the head to the knees. Then press your feet into the ground and inhale, sweep your hands out to the sides and come back to standing with your hands touching above the head, bending the knees if necessary. Exhale, take your hands down the front of your body, returning to mountain pose (tadasana) with the hands in prayer pose (anjali mudra).

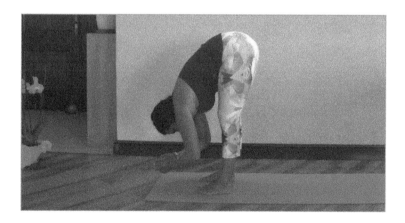

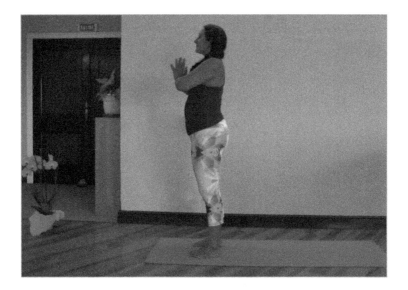

Inhale and repeat the whole sequence on the left-hand side.

After you have completed both sides, stand at the front of your mat in mountain pose (tadasana) and take a moment to check in with how you are feeling. Notice your breath, your heartbeat and your emotional state. If you are feeling well, repeat the sun salutation a few times.

Once you have become confident in doing your sun salutations, you could gradually work your way up to doing 12 rounds, that is, six each on both sides. Start by doing the first four times (two on both sides), slowly spending a few breaths in each position and then increasing the pace for the next six times. Then, for the final two sides, do the exercises slowly again, feeling the stretch and letting the heartbeat slow down.

Once you have finished the sun salutations, rest in a pose called corpse pose (shavasana; see page 76, Chapter 4).

The sun salutation has many benefits, and studies have shown that it is good for cardiovascular fitness, it strengthens muscles and joints, it can help with sleep, and it is good for anxiety. The coordination of breath with movement helps to stimulate neural pathways.

THE ART OF TRUE RELAXATION

I often ask people what they do to relax, and common replies I get include, 'Having a drink with my friends' and 'Watching television'; however, neither of these are true relaxation. Drinking alcohol can contribute to dementia and excessive consumption of alcohol can, in fact, lead to a specific alcohol-related dementia. Even drinking in moderation can affect sleep quality and the functioning of our hearts, which can, in turn, increase the risk of a stroke or a heart attack. Often when we watch television the programmes are dramatic or violent and make us feel excited, thereby stimulating our stress hormone. This is known as 'empathetic stress' and it is the stress we feel when we see someone we know or a character we identify with in danger.

True relaxation is when the mind is soft and free from tension or anxiety. There are many ways to achieve it, for example, many people might find it through a physical activity such as swimming, walking or gardening. These types of activity take the mental focus away from our thoughts. However, imagine if you had a free pass to take you into a state of true relaxation whenever you wish. Well, the good news is that you do, and it is called the breath. This book contains many ways of using the breath to relax. As you become aware of the breath, try to follow its rise and fall. If you notice that your mind is racing off somewhere else, see if you can gently bring it back to observing the breath. This form of relaxed concentration is also one of the first steps to meditation.

INTERRUPTED BREATH, VILOMA PRANAYAMA

To first learn interrupted breath (viloma pranayama) we need to be familiar with the three-part breath (see page 61, Chapter 4). Viloma pranayama is a breathing exercise that literally means 'against the grain' because it goes against or interrupts the natural flow of breath. This breathing practice helps to tone and control the muscles involved in breathing such as the diaphragm and the intercostal muscles (those between the ribs). We have seen the benefits of slow and deep breathing in Chapters 2 and 3, and this exercise helps us to control and direct the breath. This exercise can be combined with the journey of awareness exercise on page 131, Chapter 8. Make any observations about the practice in your notebook.

To perform interrupted breath (viloma pranayama), first sit in any comfortable seated position on a chair or cross-legged on the floor. In this breathing practice we work on interrupting the breath, or taking the in-breath in three stages. If three stages are too much or if the breath feels tense or restricted, always return to a normal, natural breath.

a) Start to observe your natural breath, taking five to ten full and deep breaths.

b) Take a sip of breath into the belly, and pause. Then take another sip of breath into the chest, and pause. Next, breathe all the way up to the collarbones. Pause, and then allow your exhale to be long and deep. Repeat this three to five times. Next, return to a natural breath for a few breath cycles.

c) Take a long inhale and then let the breath out in three stages, from the top of the lungs to the bottom, taking a short pause in between each stage. Repeat this three to five times. Then take a few rounds of normal breath.

d) Finally, if you feel fine, combine (b) and (c) above by interrupting the breath on the inhale and the exhale. It can be helpful to visualise you are blowing up the balloon of your lungs, and then letting the air out slowly.

After you have finished the breathing exercise, take a few deep breaths and observe how you are feeling.

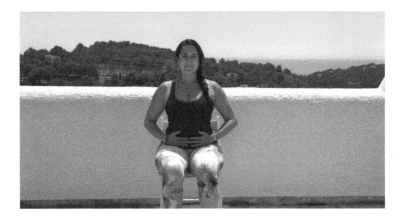

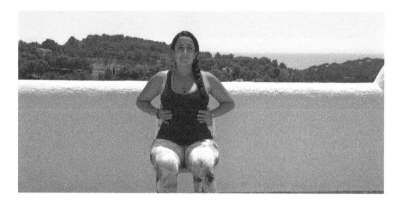

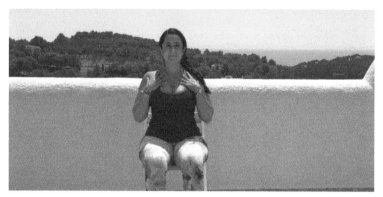

CONCLUSION

In this chapter we have explored both active physical positions and sequences that involve stretching and stimulating the body and mind. I have also provided yoga exercises that involve using sounds and mudras. The vibrations of these sounds help to stimulate the inner body and the mind, and the mudras help to practise coordinated movement. The breathing and chanting exercises involve learning relaxed concentration and focus.

I recommend you take your time to give all of these exercises a try, and then introduce some of them gradually into your daily routine. For example, you might like to practise sun salutations two or three times a week, and these can help meet recommended activity targets. The breathing exercises are great before going to bed, and a chanting exercise such as kirtan kriya is fantastic in the morning.

As with all of the exercises, write down what you do. This will help you remember the sequences and will also help you track the benefits and see which exercises are working for you, and those you are working with or caring for.

CHAPTER 10

EXERCISES FOR ANGER MANAGEMENT

Whether we have received an early diagnosis of dementia or are working with someone in the early stages of dementia, it is likely that they or we are experiencing sadness and anger. This is completely understandable as finding out we, or someone close to us, has dementia is likely to bring feelings of shock, hopelessness, regret, dismay or anger, particularly if it is our life partner who has been diagnosed. You might be asking yourself 'Why me?' or 'Why my partner/father or mother?' Many people I have met through my Yoga for Dementia project tell stories of how, after working hard all their lives, they were looking forward to an active retirement and had lots of plans for the future. Dementia, like many diseases, can feel grossly unfair, especially when we have lived healthy and active lives. You may also feel grief for the lost opportunities that you believe will accompany your, or your relative's, disease. Feeling angry is therefore a natural and normal reaction, and it is helpful to express that anger. However, when we, or others, become consumed with anger, it is not helpful for anyone.

Long-term anger can weaken our immune system and lead to health problems such as headaches, anxiety, depression, heart attack, stroke or insomnia. This is because when we are angry, our body has an emotional and physiological reaction. Anger causes our glands to produce stress hormones such as adrenaline and cortisol; this gives us a burst of extra strength, which may be good if we are getting ready to fight or flight. However, these hormones also redirect blood flowing to the stomach and intestines to the muscles instead, which is one of the reasons why stress and anger can cause digestive problems.

Anger doesn't come from the rational part of the brain; it comes from the limbic system, which is an ancient part of the brain that controls our basic emotions such as fear, and drives such as hunger. Anger arises when we feel that we cannot control certain situations or feel powerless or attacked. It can occur when certain triggers happen, or as a result of hearing bad news. Some anger can be very real, for example, when we are directly threatened. However, some anger can be as a result of the mind interpreting things in a certain way, or a misunderstanding. When we feel anger it is often useful to examine its causes. It is often our own selves and our expectations that create anger. For example, we might have been expecting somebody to do something for us, and then they did not do it and we became angry. However, it was not the person who 'made us angry' – we became angry because somebody did not meet our 'own' expectations. Those expectations and assumptions belong to us. Anger often stems from people, or society, not doing things the way we expect them to. Our expectations are based on our own culture and education, and not everyone will share the same expectations. Therefore, when we have expectations, we should look at them and maybe think about how we can better communicate those to others. There is a common Zen saying, 'No one makes you angry. You make yourself angry.'

When we are angry we should also take a pause and notice what it feels like to be angry. How do these feelings manifest within us? Do we notice ourselves getting hot? Does our heartbeat increase?

The body's stress response is interesting, as it doesn't distinguish between the first time we experienced direct anger, or when we recall it in our minds, or tell someone about an incident that made us angry. This, linked with the mind's ability to dwell on negative experiences, can result in one incident of anger being reproduced and magnified. Anger attacks our own body, so by feeding and perpetrating anger, we are really hurting ourselves. And if we are angry all the time, this can affect those around us as well, especially if we find our anger turning to aggression and we start to lash out at other people.

Yoga and meditation have been shown to be very effective in dealing with anger and can help us control our limbic system. For example, many prisoners with long histories of violence and anger have found yoga and meditation to be a great way of learning to deal with their anger and to change deeply ingrained patterns of behaviour (Bilderbeck *et al.* 2013).

In order to deal with anger, we first need to understand what anger is and how it manifests in ourselves. Everyone is different; for example, when living in family environments, we might have certain anger triggers such as someone forgetting something or continuing a bad habit we dislike. Therefore one of the first things we will practise is a meditation on anger, to understand it more fully.

ANGER MEDITATION

In this meditation we will learn to understand our anger and how it feels. This will help us realise that like all emotions, anger comes and goes, especially if we let it.

First, sit in a comfortable position with your spine straight, your hands resting comfortably, your neck straight, and your eyes gently closed. Make a commitment to yourself that you are going to focus on your feelings of anger and try to understand these feelings better.

Take a few long deep breaths to settle into the position. Then take your mind back to a recent time when you experienced anger. It is best to choose a moderate experience and not one that was too extreme. Try to remember what happened, and allow yourself to feel the anger again. Allow the feeling to grow, but not too much. Other feelings might arise as you remember that time, such as sadness or fear, but see if you can remain focused on the feeling of anger for now. Try to forget about what caused the anger, and only remain focused on the physical feeling of being angry.

Now try to really explore the feeling of anger with your awareness. Where do you feel the anger – is it in your belly, or your chest? Also, how does the anger feel – is it hot or cold? Try to visualise your anger as a ball of red or cold blue light.

Keeping this visualisation in mind, try to bring your breath into the angry feeling and imagine you are breathing directly into that angry place. Just try to be aware of the feeling of the anger and the breath going into it.

Keep going with this practice until you feel that you 'can sit' with your anger. Feel as though you are getting to know it, and making friends with it. Feel as if you are turning towards your anger, and going with it, rather than fighting against it.

Next, try to bring compassion to your anger. Anger is a normal part of being human and we all experience it. Try to observe what happens to the anger when we sit with it and experience it without reacting – does it lessen?

Next, say goodbye to the feeling of anger. Bring your attention back to your breath. Let your emotions settle down and observe how you are feeling.

After the meditation, take some time to reflect on your experience. Could you notice the anger as a particular feeling arising in your body? Were you able to accept the feelings of being angry without responding? Did you have any clarity about what is triggering your anger, any changes you could make to reduce the likelihood of it happening again, or how to better express your feelings to someone else?

Doing meditations on feelings such as anger or sadness are extremely important ways of getting to know ourselves or our friends or clients better. Many people avoid difficult emotional states by perhaps watching TV or using alcohol as a distraction. Being able to observe our reactions when we are angry, but in a safe place where we are not able to lash out, enables us to better understand when something is threatening to make us angry, and to learn how to deal with it.

This anger meditation is also particularly good for those working in caring roles, and can be adapted from an individual exercise to one that could be done together with a friend or a carer by asking the questions above in a calm environment.

We now go on to learn some active exercises that can help when we feel angry.

WOOD CHOPPING, KASHTHA TAKSHANASANA

The wood chopping exercise is a fantastic practice for releasing pent-up energy and frustration. It can be done from three positions: (a) sitting in a chair with the legs apart; (b) standing with the legs wide; or (c) squatting (for those who have practised yoga before or who are very comfortable in this pose).

Interlace the fingers and keep the palms firmly together, and sit with your back straight. Imagine the thing you are angry about or the feeling of anger on a chopping block in front of you.

Next, inhale, and take your arms straight above you, with your forearms by your ears.

When you are ready to exhale, swiftly bend forwards at the waist and take your arms down, making a strong 'haaa' sound as you exhale. The moving is like axing a tree, or swinging the arms down – hence the name 'wood chopping'.

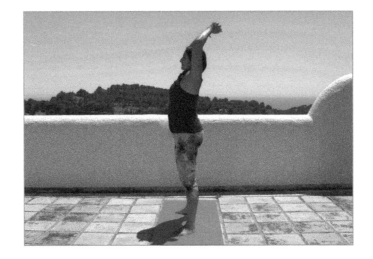

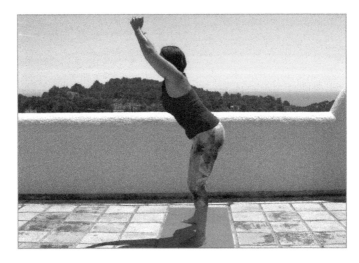

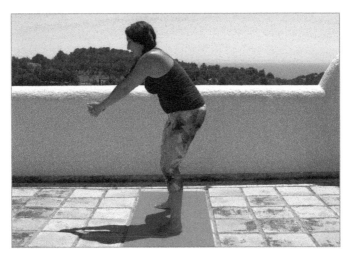

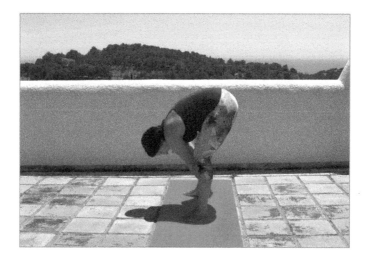

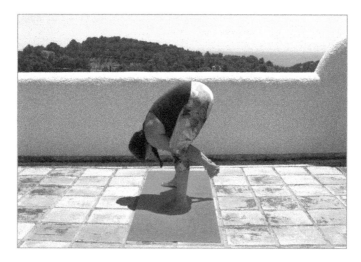

Repeat the exercise 5–15 times, building up strength and stamina each time you do it. You will probably find after doing the exercise a few times that your heartbeat will have increased, and you might feel a bit warmer.

At the end of the exercise, rest back in your chair or lie down in corpse pose (shavasana) (see page 76, Chapter 4). Then, when your breath has returned to normal, sit up slowly and take a few minutes to write down what you did and how this exercise made you feel.

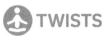 **TWISTS**

Often when we are angry we feel the anger in our belly and solar plexus. It was believed by early Buddhist monks that certain twisting poses would help release anger. Twisting poses can help to massage the internal organs and improve blood flow around the spine.

Standing twist

An easy and fun twist to do is a simple standing twist. Start by standing in mountain pose (tadasana) (see page 161, Chapter 9), then spread your legs a bit wider, turning your toes out slightly so you have a firm base to your pose.

Next, bend your knees a little and start gently twisting your torso from side to side. As you twist to the right, bring your left hand up to tap above your right chest (just below the collarbone), take your right hand behind your back to gently tap the back of your waist to the left of your spine (around where your kidneys are).

Next, twist slowly around to the other side, swinging your arms in the opposite direction and allowing your arms to gently tap the other way. Start slowly and then see if you can eventually time the movement with the breath by inhaling to the centre and exhaling to the twist. Gradually make the movements quicker, finding a good rhythm. Listen to the hands gently tapping the upper chest and kidneys. Body tapping brings many benefits and also helps to stimulate circulation.

Continue the movements for a few minutes and then slow them down to come back to the centre gradually, but do not suddenly stop. Once you come back to mountain pose (tadasana), see if you can notice any feelings within the body. You might feel slightly warmer and your heart rate might have gone up. If you feel fine, continue to the next exercise; if you feel tired or at all faint, lie down for a while in corpse pose (shavasana).

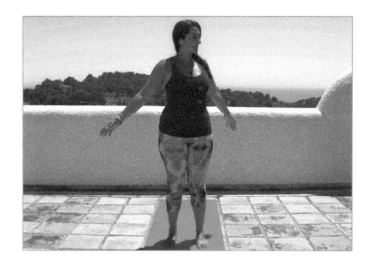

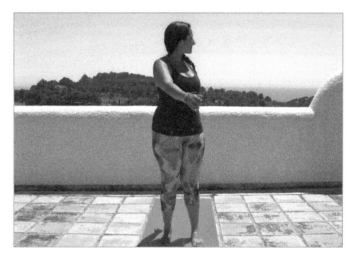

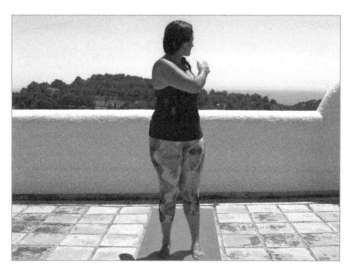

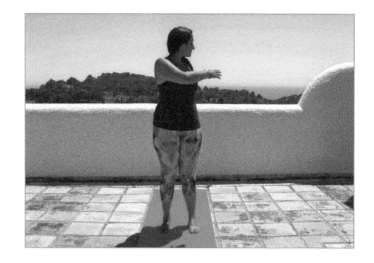

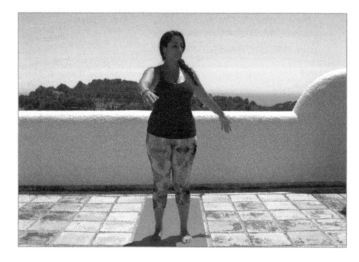

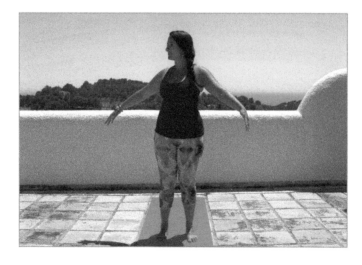

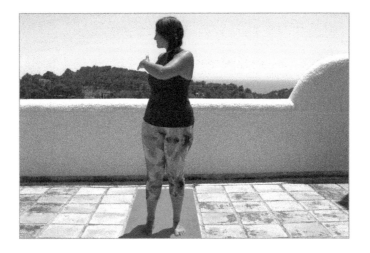

Seated half-twist

If you feel comfortable with the standing twist you will have warmed up your spine and you can attempt the next seated half-twist. This twist is ideally done from sitting on the floor, but if you would like to do this twist in a chair, see page 141, Chapter 8.

Staff pose, dandasana

This is called staff pose (dandasana), as your body is strong and straight, like a staff.

To do staff pose, start in a base position by sitting on a cushion or rolled-up blanket, making sure your bottom is slightly higher than your knees. Your spine should be straight and your legs outstretched. Take your hands to the floor either side of your spine, fingers facing forwards and palms down. Press down gently on the floor either side of your bottom and feel your spine lifting, nice and tall. Draw your shoulders back and feel the front of your chest broaden.

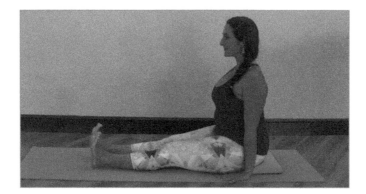

Now bring your attention to your legs. Stretch your legs out in front of you, making sure they are straight. Squeeze the legs together and flex the feet by pulling your toes towards you. Make sure your legs are engaged and you are using all your muscles.

Next, engage your belly by gently pulling your navel back towards your spine, and lift the pelvic floor by squeezing the base of the body.

Make sure your head is central on the spine; lift the crown of the head towards the ceiling. Next, gaze down at your nose and breathe slowly and deeply.

Half-twist pose

This next pose is not suitable if you have a back or spine injury.

From staff pose (dandasana), bend your right knee and place the foot flat on the floor, close to your left knee.

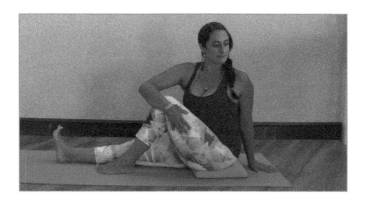

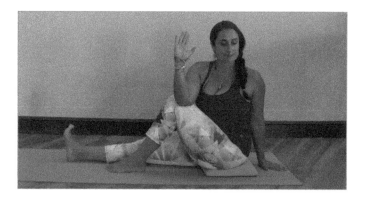

Next, lift your left hand and take it over your right knee. Hold it gently to the outside of the right knee. Lift your right hand and take it behind you on the floor. Place it with the fingers turned backwards so they point away from your bottom and your arm is straight.

As you inhale, imagine your spine growing up straight and tall, and as you exhale, try to twist a bit further, turning behind you. If your back feels fine, move your left hand further along the right thigh, hugging the thigh in to increase the twist.

Finally, if it is comfortable for you, turn your head over your right shoulder and look out of the corner of your right eye. Stay in this pose for three to ten breaths.

When you are ready to come out of the pose, start by turning your head back to the front, then your shoulders and torso back to the front.

Return to staff pose (dandasana) for a few breaths, before repeating the pose on the other side.

 BACKBENDS

Backbends are considered to be useful to tone and lengthen the spine, and help increase blood flow around the diaphragm and spine. They are particularly good for boosting mood, increasing energy and making you feel more open to new experiences. Backbends literally open up the front of the body that stretches the area around the heart, making more space for the front of the lungs and more space to breathe.

One of the easiest backbends to start with is to work against the wall. Stand about one foot distance from a blank wall, or the back of the door (be careful that there is no possibility of someone coming in).

Next, lift your arms up above your head and place them on the wall, palms facing forwards and fingers pointing upwards towards the ceiling. Spread the hands slightly wider than shoulder width. Press the palms into the wall, with the fingers spread and arms stretched up, then lean forwards, taking your chest and heart towards the wall.

Your hips should remain directly above your feet, and you should tilt your bottom up to increase the curve in the back. Remain here for five to ten breaths. A variation on this exercise involves swaying the hips from side to side to lengthen and stretch the lower back, or making small circles through the tailbone to work the hips.

When you have finished, stand back in mountain pose (tadasana), and take a few deep breaths. You can practise this two or three times a week, or when you feel you need to use this position.

Once you have practised the position a few times, you can work to move the feet further away from the wall, thereby increasing the bend of the back.

If you feel fine after the pose, you can continue to do another pose, or you can rest in corpse pose (shavasana). Again, take a moment to observe how this pose feels for you.

One you have practised the simple backbend against the wall and are comfortable with it, you might wish to try a backbend from lying down, such as cobra pose.

  ## COBRA POSE

First, lie face down on a mat or a blanket. Make sure your body is straight and even.

Next, squeeze your legs together and press your hips into the floor and pull in your belly. Then take your hands, palms facing down underneath your shoulders. Spread your fingers, push into the floor whilst at the same time breathing out and lifting your head and shoulders off the floor. Stay for a few breaths and then exhale and take your head back to the floor. Allow your forehead to rest on your hands. When you are ready, repeat the pose another one or two times, holding for as long as feels comfortable each time.

To finish, rest on the floor, wiggle your hips from side to side and again, observe how you are feeling.

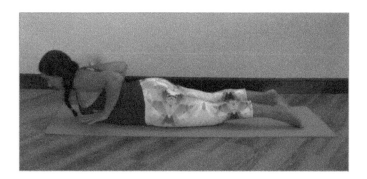

CHILD'S POSE, BALASANA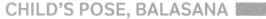

Once you have finished the backbends, take a restorative child's pose. Child's pose is a great pose for helping us turn our attention inward. It can also be very soothing if we feel that the world is against us. To perform child's pose, take the toes together and have the knees wider than the hips. Then lengthen your torso, so your body comes towards the floor in between your legs. You can rest your head on your hands or a pillow or cushion. As you rest in this position, see if you can imagine the breath flowing into your back.

Stay in this pose for 1–5 minutes. Once you have completed the pose, rest in corpse pose (shavasana).

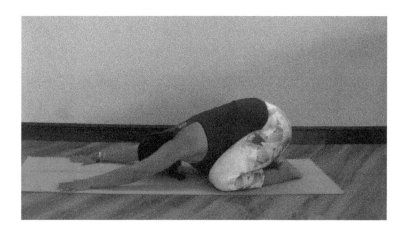

LION'S BREATH, SIMHASANA

Another fantastic traditional exercise for managing anger is lion's breath or simhasana. To do lion's breath we can either sit in a kneeling pose with the front of one foot crossed over the sole of the other foot, sitting on our heels, or sit in any cross-legged pose, or on a chair.

Imagine the object of our anger or our anger itself in front of us. Really visualise that anger or object – you could visualise it as a colour or a symbol.

Next, place your hands on your knees and really spread out and stretch your fingers wide, so they are like the claws of a lion.

Take a deep full breath in, then exhale with an open-mouthed 'haaaa' sound, like a roar, whilst at the same time taking your gaze up to the space in between your eyebrows, sticking your tongue as far out and down as it will go. Making the 'haaaa' sound helps to open the throat and release tension from the jaw. It also helps to forcibly expel air that results in deeper and fuller inhales.

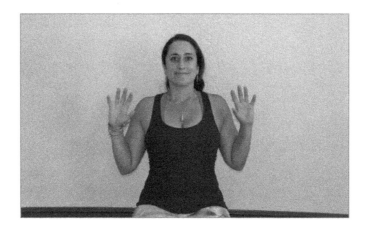

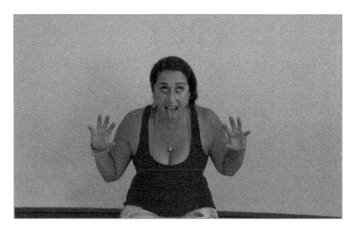

If you are doing lion's breath with a group, it is bound to cause a few laughs, and it can be a great icebreaker. When practising with a group or an individual, you can say that some people think it is a bit silly, but do encourage people to give it a try and see what the benefits are for themselves. Try it three to four times initially, and build up to more times. Really see if you can imagine that you are roaring at the object of your anger or frustration.

After completing the exercise a few times, rest with your eyes closed for a few breaths and observe how you feel, both physically and mentally.

COOLING BREATH, SHEETALI PRANAYAMA

Lion's breath is fantastic for when we feel really angry as it helps to release tension immediately. However, if we are feeling a little bit tense, or we feel we are starting to get angry, we can practise a cooling breath as a rescue remedy. This can be fantastic to do together with a client as we notice they are getting tense, or for ourselves when we feel anger emerging. There are many benefits of breathing together with a friend or a loved one, as outlined in Chapter 3.

The word sheetali comes from an ancient Indian word that means soothing or cooling. This practice has many benefits including being very calming and helping reduce stress. It can also help lower blood pressure and it is very effective for those with hyperacidity, which can be a side effect of anti-inflammation drugs. It can have a positive effect on the endocrine glands that control the release of hormones in the body and nervous system. It is also said that this practice helps to counter the effects of ageing and stimulates the whole parasympathetic nervous system (Goel n.d.).

Sit in any comfortable seated pose – cross-legged or on a chair is fine. In order to do this practice you need to roll your tongue in a little circle so it has a space in the middle, like a straw. The ability to be able to do this with the tongue is genetic, so, if you are unable to do this, take your tongue to the back of the top teeth and suck in cool air by breathing in through the mouth.

Make sure you are comfortable, then start inhaling through the mouth through the rolled-up tongue, or sucked in through the gap between the tongue and the teeth. Feel the cool air passing via the tongue. Initially inhale through the tongue for 4 seconds, and then exhale for 6 seconds through both nostrils.

Continue this practice for about 5 minutes. Then rest with a normal breath, and see how you feel.

If you enjoy this practice and feel it is beneficial, increase the breath count to 4 seconds for your in-breath and 8 seconds for your out-breath. Then, if this is comfortable for you, increase to a ratio of 5:10 and then 6:12.

If you already have low blood pressure, be careful with this breathing exercise (pranayama) as it may help to lower it further. As with any breathing exercise, if you feel that your breath is tight or you are not getting enough air, just return to a natural breath. And if you feel at all dizzy, stop doing the practice and return to normal breathing.

GANESH MUDRA, HELPING TO OVERCOME OBSTACLES

As explained in Chapter 4, mudras are a hand or body gesture that helps us direct our internal energy in a certain direction or way. We could almost see them as a type of internal body language, that is, a body language that we send ourselves. While you might feel sceptical about mudras, with all of the practices outlined in this book they are optional. But I would encourage you to try them, or help someone else to try them, before observing any results and deciding which practices benefit you or others.

Ganesh mudra helps to remove obstacles. Ganesh is a yogic deity that is considered to be a remover of obstacles. Ganesh is depicted as being a half-man and half-elephant, and when we think of Ganesh we can think of an elephant sweeping away trees and other things in its path. So, when we think about an angry elephant, maybe it can remind us to perform the Ganesh mudra.

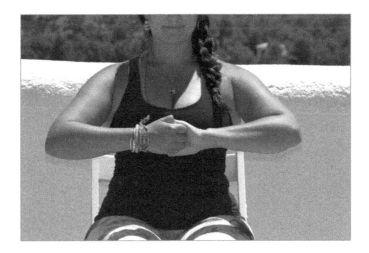

It is said that this mudra helps us overcome obstacles such as anger, and it is also said to help lift our spirits and strengthen our resolve. This mudra can also help us gain confidence. On a physical level it helps stretch and tone the cardiac muscles, which is great for getting more blood flowing to the brain. It helps strengthen the muscles of the chest, shoulders and arms. It can also help us release pain and tightness from the chest and shoulders.

Sit or stand in any comfortable position. Bend both of your elbows out to the side of your chest and turn your left palm outward so your thumb faces down and your right hand inwards, with your thumb turned up. Your hands should be about chest height. From here, bend the fingers of your right and left hand, and clasp the fingers on the right and left hand together.

Inhale, and then, as you breathe out, try to pull your arms apart while resisting, keeping your fingers locked together. As you pull the arms apart you should feel the muscles of the chest working. Resist the pull of your arms with your hands and take a few breaths. Release as you breathe out and then repeat.

At first try this mudra one or two times, gradually building yourself or those you are working with up to six times a day for best results. Again, write down how you feel, or how your clients react after performing this mudra.

CONCLUSION

In this chapter we have explored a number of methods that can help to calm us, or the people we care for, when we are feeling angry or frustrated. As I have explained in previous chapters, yoga provides a wonderful tool kit. This chapter contains a complete sequence of exercises, and you can choose to practise the whole chapter. Or, what I recommend is using bits of the chapter at a time, for example, start off with one breathing method – either lion's breath or the cooling breath – and then the simple twist and backbend. Then, as you, or the people you are practising with, progress, you can increase the level and try the other poses. Again, observation and awareness is key to reducing anger and helping with anger management, so do use the meditation on anger as a regular part of the practice.

CHAPTER 11

EASY JOINT RELEASE SERIES FOR EVERYONE, ADAPTED TO A CHAIR

This chapter introduces the first part of a simple joint release sequence and the practice of karma yoga. Both of these practices are suitable for everyone. After I completed my first yoga teacher training I went to study and spent some time living in a yogic ashram, a place dedicated to those living according to yogic principles. This experience really opened my eyes to the wider dimensions of yoga that go far beyond the modern focus of yoga as an asana-based (physical position) system.

During the time I spent living at the ashram I explored karma yoga (also known as the yoga of action), meditation, yoga nidra (yogic sleep) and very gentle physical yoga. In the ashram we always began the day with a calming joint releasing sequence. Whilst working with people living with dementia I found that an adapted version of this sequence was very effective. The great thing about this sequence is that it can be done by all people and is beneficial for all. It is wonderful for carers and family members as the gentle movements help to release tension, but it is also highly beneficial for those living with all stages of dementia. In my experience, even those with limited movements can join in some of the movements in these sequences and enjoy them. However, before I go on to explain the physical aspects of the yoga practice, I would like to talk a bit more about karma yoga.

KARMA YOGA

Yoga is not necessarily what we do on a yoga mat – it is possible to bring a yogic approach to everything we do. Karma yoga is known as the 'yoga of action', or the 'yoga of skilful action'. Now you might say, 'What do you mean by the yoga of action?' Whatever we do in our lives, for example, travelling to work, preparing food, helping others, being a mother or a daughter, talking to colleagues etc., we can do in a number of ways. Karma yoga is about seeing the wider picture of our actions, and doing them to serve others in a calm and peaceful way. When we engage in karma yoga, all of our actions become part of our yoga practice.

We can apply skilful action to all we do. So, for example, if we resent the job we are doing, or feel that we have limitations due to our illness, we might feel angry when doing them. In the ashram, everyone had to do an hour's communal work each morning, ranging from cleaning the yoga room, chopping up vegetables or cleaning bathrooms. At first I was very adverse to the idea of cleaning bathrooms, and each morning, when people were picked for tasks, I would find myself mentally resisting the cleaning activities. However, one day I was picked to do this activity and I found myself feeling very negative towards it, the ashram and myself for choosing to volunteer in the first place. To be honest, I felt fed up and wanted to go home. However, once I started the job I was paired up with a friend, the hour went fast, and I actually quite enjoyed the task. What I learned from this was that my resistance was based on my ego saying, 'I am too good for this task', and my mind telling me 'Oh you won't enjoy that.' However, once I stopped listening to my ego, I did enjoy the task. Therefore, whatever we are doing, whether it be helping someone do yoga or another action, let us see if we can use a karma yoga approach to it. Try to see an activity as a whole and part of a bigger picture, being mindful and focused in our activities, and try avoiding or ignoring mental resistance.

  ## KARMA YOGA MEDITATION

This is a meditation/mindfulness activity that you can do when doing any routine task such as brushing your teeth or making a cup of tea or helping someone you care for. It is suitable for those living with all stages of dementia (although they might need some help doing it) and for those caring for them.

Choose an everyday action, and when you are doing it, commit to watching your mental chatter. If you are unsure of what I mean by mental chatter, or find it difficult to narrow down your focus to one aspect, review the journey of awareness exercise on page 131, Chapter 8. Next, see if you can listen to this mental chatter for a while – are you enjoying the task, or are you adverse to the task? Are you focused on it or is your mind distracted?

After observing how you are doing the task, see if you can then narrow down the focus so, for example, if you are getting dressed, see if you can be very aware of all aspects of getting dressed and let your whole mind be focused on getting dressed. Think about the motivation behind your action, for example, 'I am getting dressed so I can go and enjoy this day fully', 'I am choosing or helping someone choose appropriate clothes for today.'

If you are helping somebody eat, see if you can really have your full attention on that person, their face and eyes. See if you can bring your complete awareness to the meaning of what you are doing, for example, 'I am helping someone get the nourishment they need to live.'

Whether you are yourself living with dementia or helping someone who is living with dementia, using our everyday activities to practise karma yoga has many benefits. For example, when we do activities with focused concentration, the activities are likely to be more successful. One of the early signs of dementia is forgetting how to do day-to-day activities, and using focused concentration can help. Furthermore, if you are a carer or a family member, using a karma yoga approach can help us relate to the person as an individual. So, for example, we could choose an activity to do together such as helping someone wash or moisturise their hands as our karma yoga for the day.

In yogic terms things we can do to ease the suffering of others can be one of the most rewarding roles we can do. Yes, it can also be frustrating, but only if we let the mental chatter tell us 'we should be somewhere else', or 'this is not what I intended to be doing at this point in my life' or whatever other stories we tell ourselves. See if you can let compassion come through, know that one day the roles might be reversed and someone might be caring for you, and see if you can give the precious human life you are caring for the attention they deserve.

The sun shines down, and its image reflects in a thousand different pots filled with water. The reflections are many, but they are each reflecting the same sun. Similarly, when we come to know who we truly are, we will see ourselves in all people. (Ammachi n.d.)

ENERGY-RELEASING SERIES

The next two sequences (joint release and exercises to strengthen the abdominal region) are very gentle series of poses that can have great positive effects on a number of physical disorders, and can also help our mental health and wellbeing. The poses and movements should be practised slowly with focused concentration, which is extremely helpful for developing our inner awareness and also our sense of the body's location in space. When someone is living with dementia, they often become very absorbed in their inner world, as often the outer world feels very confusing. This practice helps them use simple movements as an engaging form of activity, which gently stimulates both the mind and body.

In the ancient Indian language Sanskrit, these types of movements were known as the *sukshma vyayama*, which means a preparatory form of subtle exercises. They work on the deeper internal level to help to remove any blockages preventing the free flow of energy in the body and mind. For more about the energy points in the body or nadis, see page 59, Chapter 3. For many, stress and overwork often results in bad posture, emotional problems or an imbalanced lifestyle. In Chapters 1 and 5 we have seen the results of these sorts of problems on the production of hormones in the body. They can also cause physical tension resulting in the energy becoming blocked, leading to further tension and stiffness. Furthermore, chronic blockages such as those resulting in high blood pressure and cholesterol can result in joint or limb problems, organ failure or strokes. Therefore, these simple gentle exercises help to release tension throughout the body. We finish this chapter with a breathing exercise that is said to help balance the energy in the body and mind.

A key aspect to doing these exercises properly is ensuring that they are done with the right attitude and in a non-competitive manner. This way they not only relax the body, they also relax the mind. When we work with a strong connection to the breath we help to tone the subtle deep internal muscle groups, which in turn help to massage the organs. Furthermore, doing the exercises with long deep breathing helps to stimulate the rest and restore hormones. Combining movements with breath, and coordinating the left and right side of the body, helps to stimulate the mind, and train the fine motor skills.

In this chapter we explore those movements that help the joints, and those that help stimulate the digestion and abdominal muscles. In the next chapter we go on to further exercises that help release blocked energy. All of these sequences and breath work can work together in tandem to facilitate a free flow of energy around the body. However, if you, or those you are working with, are short on time, they can be done in separate sections. These poses can be done as often as you like, and, in fact, a little practice from each sequence each day will lead to the most beneficial effects.

SOME NOTES FOR PRACTISING AND TEACHING THE JOINT RELEASE SEQUENCE

When we first start learning yoga we might be more concerned with the outer layers of the body such as the big movements of the arms and legs and the shapes the poses make. However, yoga is about moving our awareness inwards and focusing on the inner layers.

To practise yourself or to encourage people you are working with to practise properly, ensure that you regularly stress the importance of moving with awareness. Sometimes the simpler movements are the ones that it is hardest to apply this principle to. For example, when you are doing a simple movement, watch the mind. Are you thinking of what you will be doing later, or perhaps your mind is worried about something you have been preoccupied with? Therefore the first stage when practising is to ensure that you are absorbed in the movement. Watch where the movement is starting from, which muscles you are using. If you are moving your feet, can you feel any corresponding movement in the legs and thighs? If you are moving your hands and fingers, can you feel movements in the forearms and shoulders? Can you take your mind inside your body and imagine the impulses sent by your mind to originate the movements? Can you focus your mind on the counting of the repetitions of the movements? If you are teaching a group these movements it is nice to encourage them to count the movements with you. This helps them to focus. If you notice people moving very quickly try to encourage them to slow down the movements.

Once you have practised a few times, see if you, yourself, or those you are working with can really focus on timing the movements with the breath. When the movements are timed with the breath they become slower and more controlled. This encourages the fine-tuning of the neurological processes (the workings of the brain) and greater relaxation. It is particularly beneficial to combine the movements with a light ujjayi breath (see page 65, Chapter 4).

Regular rests

When practising this series it is important to include lots of periods of rest in between each few movements. This helps us to see the effects of the movements on the part that has moved and also the breath. If you or anyone you are practising with gets tired or out of breath, always make sure you or they take some time to rest.

JOINT RELEASE SERIES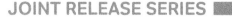

The first part of the series can be done from two positions depending on your mobility or the mobility of those you are working with. If you, or those you work with, are fairly active and can get up and down easily from the floor, start in the basic sitting position.

The basic sitting position is a bit similar to staff pose (dandasana) (see page 183, Chapter 10), but much more relaxed. Have your legs in front of you, outstretched, and your hands on the floor behind the hips, fingers pointing backwards. Support your back with your arms, but at the same time allow the body to fully relax in this position.

An alternative base position is sitting comfortably on a chair (see page 118, Chapter 7). However, in this sequence, take your hands behind you with your fingers turned back. Straighten your arms so that the spine is supported and straight. Look down your body and make any adjustments to ensure that your body is straight and even. If you are working with others, help them ensure their torso is straight. Take your spine back slightly so that the front of the body is open and you feel a nice stretch across the chest.

Toe and foot exercises

From sitting on the floor or on a chair (ideally with shoes and socks off, but these exercises can also be done with loose socks or slippers on) slowly inhale and spread the toes and stretch them towards the ceiling away from the feet; as you exhale, clench the toes together and squeeze them in towards the feet. Repeat five to ten times with a focus on the counting and the movements. If you are working with a group you could practise counting aloud; however, if you are working by yourself, focus on the internal counting.

Next, bring the awareness to the whole of the feet. If you are sitting on a chair, stretch the feet out in front of you so the heels are resting on the ground. Next, inhale and flex the feet, bringing the ankles closer to the shins, then exhale and move the feet forwards, to stretch out the front of the feet. Be aware of where the sensations are in the legs; for example, can you feel sensations in the calf muscles or shins? Repeat this five to ten times with counting. If you are working with people who find moving both legs together difficult, just work one leg at a time.

Next, we will work on ankle rotations. Using the same positions from the chair as before, with the heels on the ground, rotate the right ankle five times in one direction, then five times in the other direction, making the movement as small or as big as feels comfortable. Inhale as you bring the foot closer to the body and exhale as you take it away. Repeat the same movement with the left leg.

If your feet feel fine and you are ready to progress to the next stage, take the feet together by squeezing the whole length of the legs together. Now move the feet together in the same direction, five times in one direction and five times in the opposite direction.

Once you, or those you are working with, have practised the first two parts of the exercise a few times and are comfortable with them, you can take the legs apart and move the ankles in opposite directions. Focus on the movements travelling up the legs and the coordination of both feet moving together. Movements that synchronise the left and right side of the body are particularly good for stimulating the brain, improving our coordination and spatial awareness, which is about how we locate our body in space (see page 70, Chapter 4).

Knee exercises

From sitting on the floor or on a chair, lift your right leg, holding the leg behind the thigh. Exhale and hug the knee into the chest. As you inhale, straighten the right leg and the arms together. This is one round. Continue five times, counting with the breath. Repeat with the left leg.

Once you have practised both sides, rest for a while and check in with the breath. When you are ready to continue, lift the right leg holding, again, behind the knee, then slowly and very gently start to make small circles with the foot and shin. Inhale as you lift the shin on the top half of the circle and exhale as you lower the shin on the bottom half of the circle. Repeat up to five times clockwise and then five times anti-clockwise. Then repeat using your left leg. The knees are often prone to injury, so please ensure that you, and those you are practising with, are very careful when doing this exercise, and if there is any tweaking or pulling in the knees, rest immediately.

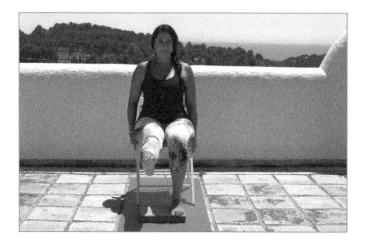

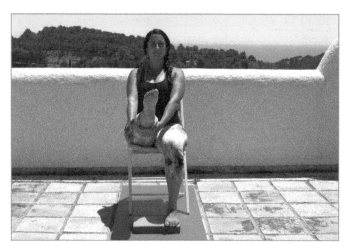

Hip openers

First, take your right leg across your left thigh. Place your right hand under your right knee to support it. Then slowly inhale to lift your right knee towards your chest and then exhale to lower it towards the floor. Use your arm and hand to support your leg at all times.

Complete five movements on the right side. Next practise the left side. Then give both your legs a shake out and relax back on the chair, checking in with how your hips feel.

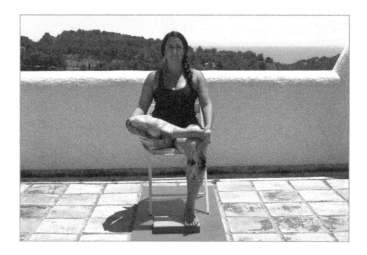

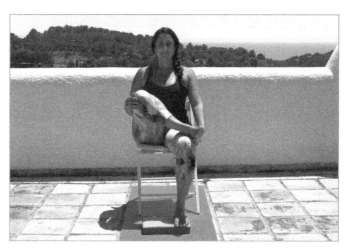

Hand movements

The hands and fingers are very important in yoga, as they are one of the most sensitive and dexterous parts of our bodies. It takes fine motor control skills to move our hands skilfully, and therefore they are one of the key parts of the body we can focus on when ourselves or someone we know is living with dementia. Also, many people living in residential care environments often no longer perform simple everyday tasks that involve using their hands, so these exercises are particularly important for improving the control of the hands. We have seen in the sections on mudras (see Chapters 4, and Chapter 14 later) that there are many reflexology points in the hands that will be stimulated by these exercises.

From any comfortable seated position inhale to open and stretch the hands and fingers wide, and exhale as you make fists with the thumbs tucked inside. Repeat this movement five times with the breath.

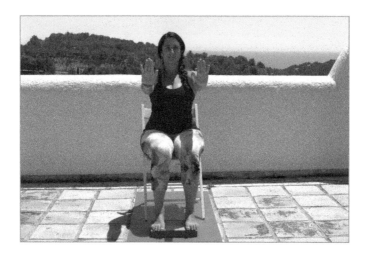

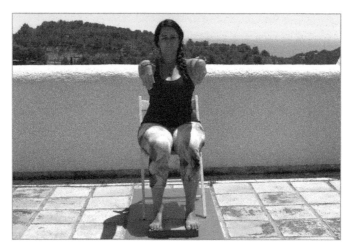

Next, stretch your arms out straight in front of you at shoulder height, open your hands and have the palms facing downwards and flat, with the fingers squeezed together. Keep your arms still, but as you inhale, move your fingers back towards your body, so you are showing the palms of your hands to the front of you (like you are making a stop sign), and as you exhale, move them down.

Focus on the feeling of the wrists and forearms working. If you, yourself, or anyone you are working with has arthritis, encourage them to do this exercise very softly, only moving according to their ability and flexing the elbows a little. They can also choose to do one hand at a time and have the fingers separate. Once you have completed the movements, rest your hands and arms down on your knees for a few breaths, with your eyes closed, and observe how your hands are feeling.

If and when you are ready, try the next exercise, which is similar to the ankle rotations we did earlier (see page 199). First, take your right arm out in front of you so it is in line with your shoulder, make a fist with the thumb inside and palm facing down. Next, make five rotations of the wrist one way and then five the other way. To finish, release the fist, give your hand a shake and rest it on your knee. Then repeat with your left wrist.

If your arms are not too tired you can then lift both arms to shoulder level, again making fists with your hands. Try moving both hands in the same direction, coordinating the movement with the breath, moving five times in one direction and five times in the opposite direction.

I recommend introducing the above two exercises first and waiting until you or the people you are working with are comfortable with them. Then, if you would like to add a challenge, take your arms in front of you again, and this time move your hands in opposite directions, five times in one direction and five times the other way. To finish, shake your hands and give them a stretch before resting them down on your knees.

Shoulder exercises

Take your arms and hands out in front of you with your arms in line with your shoulders and palms facing upwards. Exhale and bend your arms at the elbows, touching your shoulders lightly with your fingers, inhale and straighten your arms away from you. Repeat five times.

Next, keep your fingers on your shoulders but take your elbows wide and then inhale; straighten your arms so they are a 'T' shape to the body and then exhale, and bend them to touch your shoulders. Repeat five times.

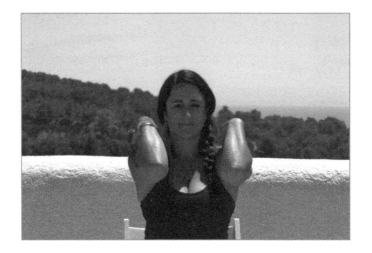

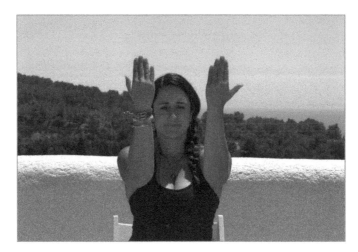

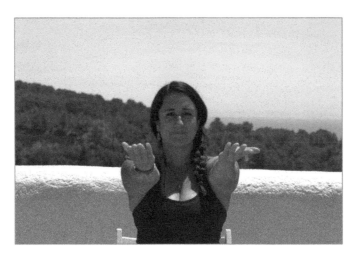

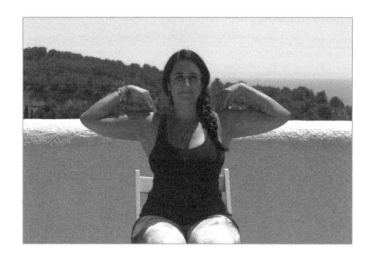

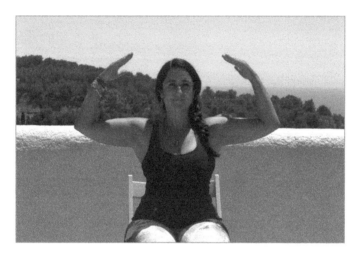

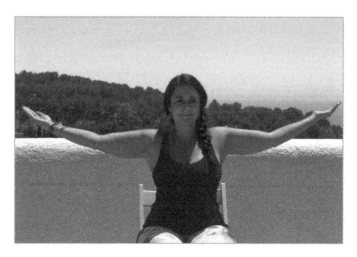

If you, or those you are working with, would like to add a coordination challenge to this exercise, you can alternate between both the above movements. So, on one inhale, your elbows move out to the front of the body, and on the next inhale, they move out to the side. After doing five of each movement, relax your hands down on your knees and take a few deep breaths.

Next, take your right fingers on to your right shoulder with your elbow out to the side. Then make five rotations in one direction with your elbow – starting small and getting bigger – and then five rotations in the other direction. Repeat with your left arm. Inhale as your arm lifts, and you create more space in the lungs, and exhale as your arm lowers.

Once you have done this exercise a few times, see if you can try both elbows together.

Neck movements

Next complete the neck movements from Sequence 2 (see page 151, Chapter 8). This sequence takes our neck through its full range of movements. The human head weighs about 4.5–5 kg, and therefore the neck often takes a lot of strain. In addition, we often hold a lot of tension in our face, neck and jaw, so these movements will help to release this.

  ## EXERCISES TO STRENGTHEN THE ABDOMINAL REGION

The next sequence of exercises aims to strength the abdominal region, which brings benefits for posture, balance, digestion and helps strengthen the pelvic floor muscles.

From sitting in a chair, straighten your right leg and inhale to raise it so it is in line with your hip, squeeze in the belly, then your pelvic floor, and hold your leg up for 2–3 seconds. Then lower your leg. Practice up to five times with the right leg and then repeat with the left leg.

Once you are comfortable with this exercise, try to do it with both legs together. However, both legs together is quite strong, so only do so if you do not have any back pain or other back issues.

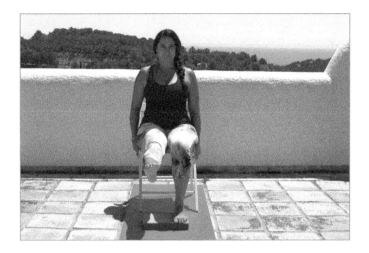

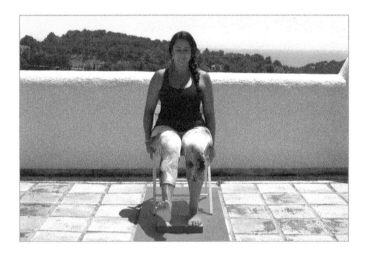

If you are comfortable with the alternate leg raises, support your body with both hands on the seat of the chair and then perform slow, controlled, cycling movements with both legs. Cycle for three to five breaths in one direction and then reverse the movement for another three to five breaths. Never strain in this movement, and if moving both legs together is too much for the coordination of the person you are working with, or yourself, first practice with one leg at a time.

After doing this movement, finish with the twists as described in Sequence 1 (see page 138, Chapter 8).

ALTERNATE NOSTRIL BREATHING, NADI SHODHANA

To finish this sequence we can try a breathing exercise called alternate nostril breathing, or nadi shodhana. As explained in Chapter 3, yoga helps to cleanse or clear out our energy channels (known as the nadis). Alternate nostril breathing is said to help balance the right and left side of the brain. Alzheimer's disease and other dementias will affect the right and left side of the brain differently, and can affect the corpus callosum, the part of the brain that connects the right and left hemispheres of the brain. Therefore exercises to stimulate both the right and left side of the brain can be beneficial for those living with dementia. Alternate nostril breathing is also said to help clear thinking and enhance our ability to concentrate, and is also great for families or carers.

Sit in any comfortable position. Spend some time checking your position is stable and your spine is straight, and then commence normal natural breathing through your nose. If you feel you need to settle in more and be more present before starting the exercise, do a few rounds of full yogic breath (see page 61).

Next, take the first two fingers of your dominant hand to your eyebrow centre and breathe in through both nostrils.

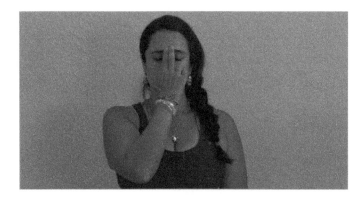

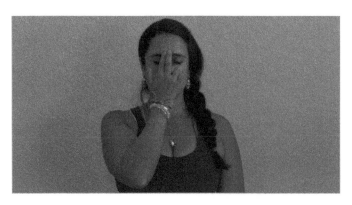

Close your right nostril with your thumb and then breathe out fully through your left nostril. When you have fully finished the out-breath, breathe in again through your left nostril and then close your left nostril with your ring finger, and breathe out of your right nostril.

Next, breathe in through your right nostril and then close your right nostril while releasing your left nostril, and breathe out of the left nostril. This is one complete round of alternate nostril breathing (nadi shodhana).

The same sequence is then repeated for each subsequent round. Inhale through the left nostril, exhale through the right nostril, inhale through the right nostril, and then finish by exhaling through the left nostril.

Practise three or four rounds to start, and gradually, over a period of weeks, build yourself up to 5 minutes a day.

Once you have finished the practice, exhale out of your left nostril. Breathe in through both nostrils and enjoy a few rounds of full yogic breath. Take a moment to notice how you are feeling, and then stretch and open your eyes.

CONCLUSION

In this chapter we have explored a very simple series of exercises. Try to practise a few at a time, remembering to always note them down in a notebook to help you remember what you have practised, and to keep track of how you feel after you have done them. As described throughout this chapter, the exercises should be done with relaxed focus and concentration. This helps to ensure we are bringing the sixth limb of yoga (dharana, or focused concentration) into our practice. Remember throughout these practices to also watch your mental chatter. When I first started doing some of the simple practices in this chapter I remember thinking they were a bit boring and I wanted to do more difficult asanas (or positions). However, after practising them for a number of weeks, I began to realise the profound benefits of doing simple movements with awareness.

STIMULATING THE SENSES

This chapter is intended to flow on seamlessly from the previous chapter, so before attempting the sequences in this chapter, I strongly recommend that you are familiar with practising or leading the sequences from the previous chapter. These poses are simple and fun, and help to stimulate the senses!

The poses in this chapter specifically work on unblocking stored or stuck energy and can be a helpful release from negative emotions. As with previous movements we have learned, such as the wood chopping exercise (kashtha takshanasana) (see page 177), they mimic natural actions, and help take the body and spine through a full range of movements.

This chapter also contains touch practices including body tapping and a gentle hand massage. Lightly tapping the body to produce a sound is a wonderful practice that helps to stimulate the blood flow and the whole body. It is particularly beneficial for those with circulation issues. Tapping is also said to help stimulate the body's energy lines, and has been used in many ancient practices such as Tai Chi.

The chapter begins with some suggestions regarding essential oils that can benefit the practice of yoga.

ESSENTIAL OILS

Yoga can be highly effective when combined with the use of natural essential oils. Essential oils are extracted from plants and flowers and are made up of the part of the flower or plant that gives it its smell. Essential oils have been used for hundreds of years and have been valued for their medicinal properties. There are many types of oil, and we explore here some common oils that can be particularly helpful for those living with dementia.

Essential oils are available in some pharmacies or can be ordered online. When ordering oil, be careful to invest in pure, natural oils.

Here is a good list of oils to start with:

- lavender and lemon balm, to reduce anxiety and agitation

- peppermint and rosemary oil, to stimulate the appetite and support memory

- bergamot, to help calm the mood, fight depression and aid sleep

- rosemary, to improve memory and cognition.

You can use aromatherapy oils in a number of ways. You can use an aromatherapy diffuser and try diffusing one type of oil at a time during your yoga sessions. I recommend starting with lavender as this is a common and recognisable scent and is generally very calming, and as it is said to lift the mood, it can also help tap into distant memories. If you or those you are working with are restless, try using lemon balm instead, which is said to be good for anxiety.

For active movements I recommend peppermint or rosemary oil. Peppermint is great to use in sessions before lunch as it is said to help stimulate the appetite. Rosemary is said to improve memory and is a good aromatherapy oil for Alzheimer's (Moss *et al.* 2008).

A great way to use essential oils is to first combine them with a base oil such as almond oil and to use them on the skin. For example, dilute a few drops of lavender oil with almond oil and use it for the hand massage described on page 221, later in this chapter. Essential oils can also be used as an aid in meditation, and one of the best ways to try this is to mix a few drops of lavender oil with a base oil and then place this on your eyebrow centre, or that of the person you are working with. This can be used during any of the guided relaxation or meditation practices. However, before starting any new seated practice, it is always beneficial to move a little bit to release any blocked energy and to help others release theirs.

A SIMPLE ENERGY-RELEASING SEQUENCE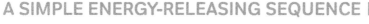

This series of poses and practices is designed to help release blocked energy in the body. It also helps to break down neuromuscular knots in the body. Neuromuscular knots are hypersensitive, pea-sized nodules that can develop in injured muscles. They can lead to muscle stiffness, tiredness and weakness. Therefore this sequence is particularly useful for those with a lack of energy and a stiff back. They also eliminate energy blockages in the spine, activate the lungs and heart and improve endocrine function. They can be done either slowly or more vigorously. However, if someone has a heart condition or other serious issues, they should always proceed with caution. These positions can be excellent for getting rid of pent-up energy and frustration that often comes with dementia.

All of the positions in this sequence can be done from sitting on a chair (as described in 'Before you begin', page 117, Chapter 7) or on the floor from a base position (as described on page 183, Chapter 10).

Pulling the rope!

Sometimes we can feel like our lives are like an uphill struggle, especially when someone we know or care for is living with dementia or we ourselves have been diagnosed with dementia. There are often many things such as care to organise, and routine tasks can take a lot longer than normal.

This exercise is great for heart health, but combining the physical exercise with a powerful visualisation can increase its emotional benefits. As we are doing this exercise that mimics pulling a rope, imagine we are pulling something we need down towards us, such as hope, love or patience. So, for example, if you need more strength, with each pull imagine you are pulling strength towards you. Before you start this exercise, think about something you need to pull down. If you are helping a group do this exercise, each choose a word and then go around the circle, each saying, 'I pull down love', 'I pull down hope' etc. If someone in the group is unable to articulate their needs, don't worry as they will benefit from hearing you and the others say the positive words.

Once you have gone round the group and all had a chance to say something, imagine there is a rope hanging down in front of the middle of your body. Breathe in and reach up high with your right hand and close your fingers, like you are holding on to a rope. As you exhale bring your hand down the centre of your body; try to create a feeling of resistance through your arms like you are pulling down a heavy rope. Follow the movement of your hands with your eyes. Once your right hand is down and resting on your knee, do the movement with your left hand. This is one round of the exercise. Repeat four to eight rounds and remember to breathe in as you lift your hand and out as you lower your hand.

Keep your awareness on your breath and time each movement with one breath. Keep your awareness on the emotional feeling you are drawing down, for example, love, hope.

Once you are familiar with the exercise, combine the physical movements with the words 'I pull down...'. This can make it both fun and dynamic.

This movement is excellent for stretching the back and shoulder muscles. If you or someone in the group you are leading cannot move both arms, or cannot lift their arms very high, they can still join in the exercise to the best of their ability.

MOVEMENTS THROUGH THE SPINE

The next two exercises help to take the spine through a range of movements including twists.

Sit in a comfortable position on a chair or on the floor. Have your legs spread a little wider than hip distance. If you or the person you are working with have no problems in the hips, spread the legs wider, up to a 90-degree angle.

On an inhale breath spread both arms wide with palms facing forwards and arms straight. Have your arms at about shoulder level.

Next, as you exhale, take your right hand towards your left toe or knee. Keep your left arm straight and if comfortable for your neck, look towards your thumb. If not, keep your head in line with your spine.

Inhale and bring the torso and head back to a central position before repeating on the other side. This is one round. To start, try about four to eight rounds. I recommend starting slowly and resting your hands down at the side of the body for one or two cycles of breath in between each round.

When you are more familiar and comfortable with the exercise you can do a few rounds and then rest for a few breaths. This exercise can also be done for more rounds with faster breathing, to make it more dynamic.

If anyone you are working with has any neck issues, do not turn the head to look at the back hand when twisting. Instead, keep the head in line with the spine.

To help with coordination, and to change the focus of the exercise, the breathing can be reversed so you breathe in as you twist and out when you return to centre. This applies more pressure to the abdomen and can help tone the abdomen and increase digestion.

As you are doing this movement, keep your focus on the breath and movement and also the twisting motion in the spine. If you or anyone you are working with has a back condition, move the spine only a little bit to each side and very gently.

Churning the mill

When I was 18 I went to see my paternal grandparents in India who lived in a small town in Punjab (an agricultural region in the north of India). The Punjab is very traditional, and my grandmother would do all her food preparation by hand. This included making homemade buttermilk that involved a churning motion. I used to help my grandmother with this chore and found the churning movements very beneficial for my whole torso and waist. Despite being in her late 70s my grandmother did all her chores including washing her clothes and sweeping the floors etc. by hand. These movements took her body through a full range of movements, which I am convinced helped her stay supple and strong.

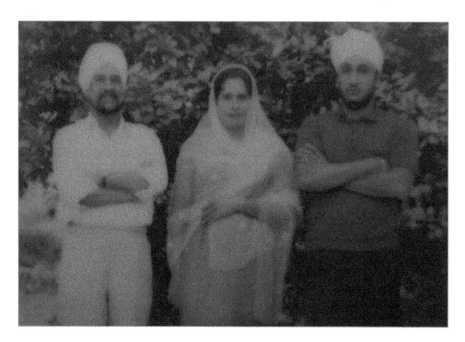

This movement can be done from sitting on the floor or on a chair and, as with the last position, the knees can be wide, and if sitting on the floor, the legs can be straight.

Interlace your fingers and stretch out your hands in front of you with your elbows straight, if possible. Inhale with you body at the centre, and as you exhale, begin to move your hands towards your right knee or foot, then move your hands over to the left knee and then back to the centre. Your hands should be drawing a big circle, like churning a mill. Inhale when you come back to the centre and if you can, lean back a little bit as this will help engage your abdominals. One rotation is one round. Try doing about four to eight rounds in one direction and then do the same number in the other direction.

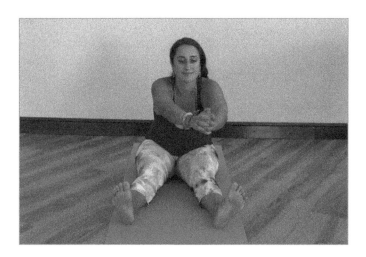

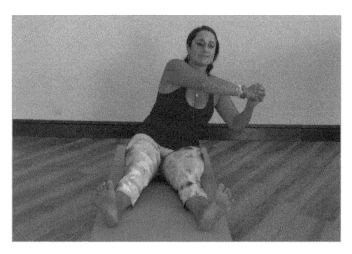

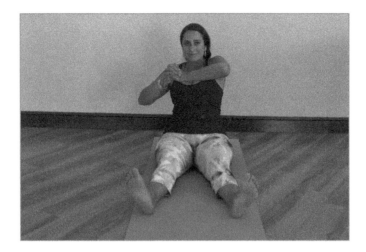

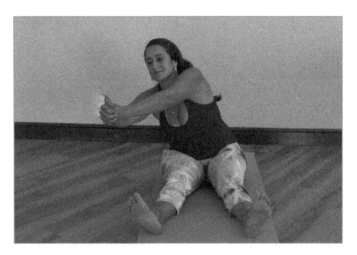

This movement is fantastic for toning the nerves and organs of the pelvis and stomach region. Once you or those you are working with are comfortable with this movement it can be varied; for example, instead of just drawing a wide circle the circle can start off small and become wider on each rotation, thereby making more of a spiral movement. This will work a wider range of muscles and also help with muscle coordination.

Picking fruit

My maternal grandmother who is now living in residential care used to have a huge garden full of fruit trees. One of her favourite things used to be to pick fruit and make jam. Fruit picking is the inspiration behind this exercise, and again, as with the pulling the rope exercise, we can imagine we are pulling down something we need into our life, for example, that we are picking down sunshine or colour. This exercise is fantastic for strengthening the muscles on the side of the body and the lateral muscles that go across the spine, which are good for balance.

From a chair or base position, start with your spine straight. Then imagine your favourite tree just above you. As you inhale, lift your right hand and arm up and stretch up, feeling as though you are picking a piece of fruit. Feel a stretch from your right fingers to your right hip. Exhale, and take your hand down. Then repeat on the left side. Repeat both sides for 10–20 breaths. Then rest with your hands down on your knees.

Rowing the boat

This exercise mimics the action of rowing a boat and is fantastic for your waist, pelvis and torso. The movement can either be done sitting on a chair (but you will need to sit forwards so you will have space to lean back), or it can be done from a base position (see page 183, Chapter 10).

Hold your hands in front of you and imagine you are holding oars with palms facing down. Take a deep breath in, and sit up straight. Then, as you breathe out, bend forwards and straighten your arms as far out in front of you as you can manage.

As you breathe in, lean back using the muscles of your waist, and bring your hands back towards your shoulders. Your hands should make a smooth circular movement. This is one round. As you move, feel as though you are stretching from the hips to the fingers on the inhale and as you move backwards, suck your belly in a little so that the movement comes from the centre of the body and not just the arms.

First try practising four to eight rounds, and then take a rest to see how the movement has affected you or those you are practising with. Afterwards you can reverse the movement and practise the same number of rounds. If you would like to introduce a fun element to this exercise you could try singing a few rounds of 'Row row row your boat gently down the stream' whilst doing it; this will help people warm up for the bhakti yoga practices (see Chapter 13). However, please be careful about doing this, as we are not aiming to be patronising. If you do introduce singing, it should be seen as being more of a fun thing to add on.

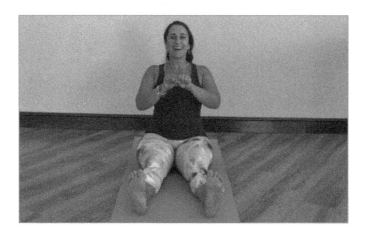

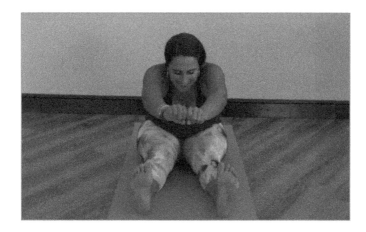

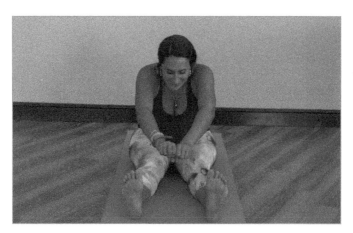

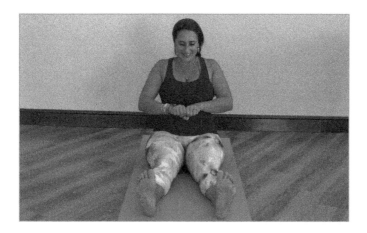

Once you are comfortable practising and teaching the first part of the exercise, you might like to attempt a variation of this exercise.

Starting from the same sitting position, spread your legs as wide as possible. If you are sitting on the floor your legs should be straight; if you are on a chair they can be bent. Turn to the right and row over the right leg as you exhale, inhale back to centre. Next, turn to the left, exhale and row over the left leg. Then turn back to the centre and row over the space between the legs or feet. This is one round; try to practise three or four rounds and gradually build yourself or those you are working with to up to six to seven rounds. As you or those you are practising with are moving, keep your gaze focused on your hands and your awareness on your breath and the movement in the lower back and pelvis area.

Wood chopping, kashtha takshanasana

As well as being a fantastic pose for releasing anger, the wood chopping exercise (kashtha takshanasana) is also great for blocked energy so it can be included in this sequence of poses. The wood chopping exercise is explained on page 177, in Chapter 10, so please take a look and perform this pose six or seven times.

After performing the wood chopping, I recommend resting for a while to see the effects of all the poses so far, and check in with how you feel. All of these poses are designed to help release energy. They can be performed slowly but also more vigorously. I recommend practising them slowly to start with, and then building up speed and pace, depending on how you, or the clients you are working with, are feeling.

These fun poses are best done in the morning or before lunch, as they tend to be invigorating. Most of the movements mimic the natural movements people do in their lives and are great at taking the body through a full range of movements. When I have worked with groups of people living with dementia they have really enjoyed making up their own movements, and this is something I encourage. Therefore you or those you are working with can think back to movements you used to do and enjoy, for example, swimming, playing the piano or trumpet, running, cycling etc., and spend a few minutes practising each.

A way to incorporate this into a fun group activity is to include a session where everyone says their name and then shows a movement. Then everyone else copies the movement for a few minutes. Helping people to make up their own movements can be great for those living with mid-stage dementia as it helps them feel empowered, and can be a great way of encouraging group bonding if you are working with a group. In addition, asking people to make up movements based on natural movements helps to increase the range of movements they can do. It is good to ask people to do the made-up movements after they have practised the movements in this and the previous chapter, as they should have a better idea about how to move with the breath. Ideally we should breathe in when we do movements that open the chest and exhale when we do movements that close the lungs.

After completing these dynamic energy-releasing positions, take a while to review how you or those you are working with are feeling.

  ## STIMULATING THE SENSES WITH TAPPING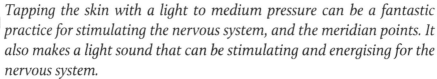

Tapping the skin with a light to medium pressure can be a fantastic practice for stimulating the nervous system, and the meridian points. It also makes a light sound that can be stimulating and energising for the nervous system.

Start by sitting or standing, and begin to lightly tap your head with your fingertips, tapping all over the head and forehead.

Next, with the first two fingers, tap from the eyebrow centre to the temples and around under the eyes. Circle the eyes a few times, lightly tapping.

Next, tap where the upper and lower jaw meet, being sure to relax the jaw at the same time.

Next, tap the back of the neck and the shoulders.

Then, using one hand, tap from the shoulder down the outside edge of the other arm and then up the inside edge of the arm. Next, tap across the front of the chest and then swap hands, tapping down the other arm.

Next, tap the upper chest, sides of torso, waist and then in clockwise circles, around the belly.

Then, using the whole hand, tap around the hips, then down the sides of the legs, then come back up, first up the inside of the legs and then up the front of the legs. Repeat a few times.

Afterwards make the hands into light fists and tap down either side of the spine from top to bottom and then down the backs of the legs. Repeat a few times.

Last, give your hands, head and legs a shake and sit still, noticing how you feel.

It has been shown that many people living with dementia will benefit from being touched in a gentle and appropriate manner; however, often caregivers might be reluctant to touch older people due to a lack of confidence. A simple 10-minute hand massage has been shown to significantly decrease aggressive behaviour and stress levels for those living with dementia (Caitlin 2015).

STIMULATING THE SENSES WITH A GENTLE HAND MASSAGE

This short massage will help build someone's trust before helping them put their hands into a mudra (see page 66, Chapter 4 and page 239, Chapter 14). First, ask the person's permission to touch their hands and then, if they seem happy by either saying yes, or through their facial expression, start by simply holding their hands. If their hands are dry, you could use a hypoallergenic unscented massage cream or any hand cream. Gently rub the lotion all over their hands whilst watching their face. Watching their face whilst you massage them will help you gauge how hard to press their hands, and will help you check they are enjoying the massage. Next, take one hand and support it in yours and give each of their fingers a series of gentle squeezes from the base of their fingers to the fingertips. Make gentle circular motions on each finger segment in between your finger and thumb. Turn the hand upwards and make small circular motions on their palm with your thumb, massaging the fleshy bit of their palm. Then, using both your thumbs, stroke the palm with downward motions. Place the person's hand gently back in their lap. Do the same sequence with their other hand.

As you are massaging the person's hands try to be really present with the person you are working with. Try to notice their hands and if their right and left hand are different, try to notice if their hands are rough or smooth. As you work with them you might like to think about the type of life they have led and the work their hands have done. Finish this hand massage by holding both their hands in yours and looking into their eyes.

SOUND EXERCISE, 'SEA OF OMS'

The word 'om' is often used in yoga. It is considered to be a powerful universal mantra, one that can be used by anyone. Om has many different meanings and it is said to be a very primal sound. Om is actually made up of three distinct sounds, a-u-m. The sounds are said to represent many things including creation, life and destruction. When done properly we can feel the sound of the om from the base of the spine to the crown of the head. The vibrational frequency of the sounds can be soothing and make us feel very tranquil.

A great way to practise om is to do it in a group to create a 'sea of Oms', which is a bit like an orchestra of 'oms' all sounding at different times and at different pitches! To teach 'sea of Oms' in a group, first start with chanting 'om' together in unison. Encourage people first to chant at a normal volume, then to chant loudly, and then softly, and practise chanting using different tones. Once the group gets into the chanting, encourage everyone to begin chanting at different times, and at different frequencies, thus creating a sea of continuous sound like an orchestra, with each person's 'instrument' or 'om' making different sounds. Remind the group that it doesn't matter if the oms are in tune or not. The main thing is to chant and feel the vibrations and the vibrations of everyone working together.

This is a great exercise to do in a group as the different sounds of the 'om's can be very uplifting; in this exercise there is also no right or wrong, so people are free to make the sounds they wish. Try to encourage people to open their mouths and feel as though the sound is coming from the back of their lungs and the pit of their bellies. Encourage people to vary chanting loudly and softly and let themselves be carried by the sound. If somebody does not want to join in the chanting or cannot, they will still benefit from listening to the others chant.

Try this first and then move on to trying a simple kirtan chanting (see page 159, Chapter 9). When chanting with a group they might at first feel a bit shy, but in my experience, after a few sessions, the groups I've worked with have loved the chanting.

CONCLUSION

It is well known that multisensory stimulation is beneficial for people living with dementia, in fact stimulating the senses has been shown to help reduce agitation and improve sleep. In this chapter we have explored a variety of ways to stimulate our senses. We have used the sense of smell via introducing natural essential oils into our yoga sessions, including those that have been shown to benefit those living with dementia. We also use a range of movements which mimic natural movement, combined with visualisations. These movements also help us and those we are working with get a sense of how fast they are moving and in what direction. We also use sound via chanting practices. In this chapter we also introduce tapping, which stimulates the senses through sound, touch and helps us develop our sense of our bodies location in space. We have explored practices we can do in a group, but also those we can do on a one-to-one basis.

CHAPTER 13

BHAKTI YOGA

In this chapter we explore bhakti yoga. Bhakti yoga is a form of practising ishvara pranidhana or 'surrendering to the divine'. In the Introduction, the fact that yoga is very much a secular practice and can be practised by anyone from any religion was discussed, or indeed, if you are an atheist (meaning you do not believe in a higher power) or agnostic (meaning that you believe in a higher power but not in a specific form). Many people in India and all over the world practise bhakti yoga, and you might have even practised bhakti yoga before without knowing it.

Bhakti yoga is considered yoga's path of love or devotion, and it is said to be one of the easiest paths of yoga to master. It is about surrendering to the divinity within our own self and recognising the unique individual life within all of us. Bhakti yoga is not about doing certain positions or breathing exercises; rather, it is about cultivating love in our hearts and developing a sense of the preciousness of life. A bhakti yogi can practice anytime, anywhere. Bhakti yoga is also a wonderful addition to other yoga practices as the things we cultivate in our bhakti practice can add flavour and colour to our other practices, thereby making them more meaningful and fulfilling.

When I was in my early 20s, before I became a yoga teacher and while I was on a trip to see my grandparents in India, I visited Rishikesh and stayed in a yoga ashram overlooking the vast and beautiful river Ganges. Many of the other people staying in that ashram with me were western and mainly interested in the asana, pranayama and cleansing practices of yoga. However, I would walk down into the town and visit the Sivananda yoga ashram. Sivananda was one of the leading teachers of yoga until his death in 1962. His style of yoga is still very popular today.

At the Sivananda ashram one evening I came across many older Indian women who must have been in their 70s and 80s. They sat in the temple singing very hypnotic and repetitive songs known as bhajans or kirtan.

These simple songs are songs about life, but also contained the theme of letting go and surrendering to the river of life. This was very poignant as the river Ganges is one of the great rivers of the world, and directly supports and influences the lives of the estimated 500 million people who depend on its water. It is also the spiritual home of yoga as it is said that it was on the banks of the river Ganges where Shiva, the mythological founder of yoga, taught yoga to his wife, and this is where yoga began. So later in this chapter I introduce some simple bhakti practices that can be done by anyone of any religion or none. My grandmother and the grandmothers of Rishikesh inspire the inclusion of these practices in this book.

Human life is a precious gift, and if we think about the special set of circumstances that led to each of us being present on the earth, from evolutionary history to our own family history, we can recognise the magic of us being here. So whether we believe in a god on not, cultivating a state of gratefulness for the gift of life can be a wonderful practice. If we believe in a form of god, whether it is Jesus, Mary, Allah, Krishna or any other 'god', we can use them as our focus in bhakti practices; if we do not believe in a specific god, we can devote our practices to the Divine, the Beloved, the Spirit, the Self, or the Source. If you, or those you are guiding, wish to practise bhakti yoga they can choose what they wish to devote their practice to, be it a person, deity, object, mountain, river or idea.

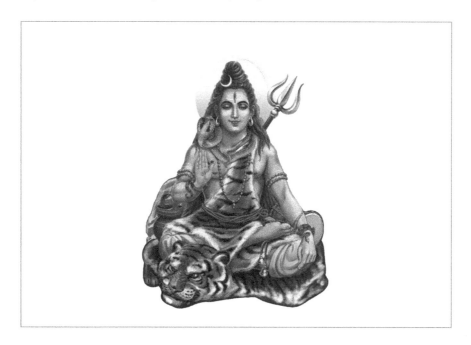

If you are not sure where to seek guidance, ask the universe for guidance on what to do, whom to devote yourself to, how to pray and when to do it. You or those you are working with may need to ask this question more than once as surrendering to bhakti yoga takes dedication and a certain letting go of the ego, which is why it is particularly useful for those living with dementia. As their memories fade and they lose a certain sense of themselves, this opens up space for the ego to lessen and for us to come closer to 'god', so bhakti yoga can act as a rock in a time of change. It can provide solace and give meaning to some of the things that happen in our lives. Coming from a not particularly religious background, I have found bhakti yoga has provided me with light in times of darkness.

Bhakti yoga can take on many forms; for example, you can use prayer, chanting or repetition of a mantra. Bhakti yoga is about creating more love in our lives, and sometimes to do so we must go through periods of pain. Having a loved one diagnosed with dementia or working with someone living with dementia can be a very painful experience. However, working with bhakti yoga can help us find ways we can use our experiences to love more, and suffering has often created much human strength, empathy and compassion for others.

Below are a number of ways to practise bhakti yoga.

SIMPLE SEATED PRACTICE, SENDING LOVE TO OTHERS AND THE WORLD

In this exercise, sit in a comfortable seated position, or you can even do it lying down. Bring to mind a person or situation in the world that needs healing – this might be a friend, or an area of the world that is suffering with war, or a family member, or animal, or the planet that is suffering. Try to have a strong visualisation of the person or situation, and then imagine you are sending healing love or energy to that person or thing. Try to imagine the hardship or peril that person is in, and see if you can send them compassion and love. You might like to imagine your healing energy as a white light, and simply focus on sending that person or situation that light. Do this for 5 or so minutes, and then notice how you feel after.

Focusing your energy on someone, or on something else other than your own situation, can be a wonderful way of putting your own problems into perspective. It can also help people get out of repetitive and negative thought patterns.

INFUSING EVERYDAY ACTIONS INTO ACTIONS OF JOY AND DIVINITY

We have a choice in the way we perform everyday actions. One way of getting more joy into our lives is to work on trying to be more present in our everyday actions and those we do with others we care for. As discussed earlier, losing our own memories can create more room for other feelings such as trust, compassion and love. Therefore, choose a routine action that you do each day, and see if you can do it with more compassion, presence and love. As educated human beings we have been born in a very privileged position and have the power of choice in how we approach tasks in our lives. So see if you can find some joy, peace and gratitude for the small actions and things in life. For example, if you are working with other people, see if you can really look at them, into their eyes and smile at them. If you have a relative visiting see if you can sit with them and simply hold their hands. How we perform the small actions in life and our mental attitude to them has a big impact on our whole life.

BEING KIND TO OURSELVES AND OTHERS

Another way to foster more love in our lives is to be kind and grateful to others. So whether we are caring for someone living with dementia or we, ourselves, are living with dementia, try to be kind. This could be via small acts such as saying thank you for deeds people help us with, or smiling and asking someone how they are, or being patient with someone when they ask you the same question multiple times. We can also write a thank you note to a colleague, pay someone a genuine compliment, or show other acts of kindness.

Try to do things that will also help to heal and nurture your relationships. So, for example, if someone has wronged you, try to see the situation through their eyes and see if you can forgive them. We are all human and all have faults and make mistakes. See if you can accept your own faults, as this will make it easier to accept and forgive the faults of others. To help with this you might want to try the loving-kindness mettā meditation on page 109, Chapter 6.

NATURE THERAPY

It is well known that nature can be a wonderful healer, and many studies have shown that nature can have positive effects on stress reduction. In the adult residential care sector this is being recognised, and more new homes are being designed with outdoor areas, sensory gardens and terraces, so people living with dementia can experience and enjoy the outdoors. Appreciating nature can also be a form of bhakti yoga and mindfulness, and many yoga practices were inspired by nature, for example, the sun salutation and poses named after animal forms. In addition, yoga nidra (see page 234, Chapter 14) also often contains natural images.

The easiest way we can use nature as part of our yoga practice is to do our practice outside. Many residential homes have outdoor areas, or, if you are practising at home, you could use an outdoor area if you have one. Or you could go to the local park. When you are practising outdoors or helping others practise outside, see if you can encourage yourself or others to really feel nature; for example, see if you can feel the sun on your face or the breeze against your skin. Focus on listening to natural sounds and encourage others to do the same. You might also like to try the four directions meditation that helps us connect with the natural elements (see page 243, Chapter 14).

Another simple practice that can be done on a walk is to pick a flower and spend some time reflecting on its beauty. The flower can then be pressed in the pages of your notebook or journal to remember that time.

SINGING OR CHANTING

One of the most common types of bhakti yoga practices is to practise singing or chanting. This can be a simple and uplifting practice, and, as described above, it does not matter if you are religious or not. First, start by listening to kirtan, gospel or any other devotional music that moves you. Once you have listened a few times, try to sing along. If you are working with a group, you could try practising some very simple kirtan such as 'Jai Mai' or 'Hey Shiva'. These types of kirtan practices help to celebrate the divine feminine and masculine principles, and you do not have to be a Hindu to sing them. There are many free versions of these chants on YouTube, but to start, try those by Krishna Das, Wah! or Snatam Kaur.

Another great healing mantra is a Buddhist-based chant, 'Lokah samastah sukhino bhavantu', or 'May all beings be happy and free'.

Before you start singing or chanting, it is a good idea to loosen up vocal chords by practising the 'sea of Oms' (see page 222, Chapter 12). This can also help people get over any shyness or reluctance to sing in a group. When chanting or singing kirtan there is no need to worry about what your voice sounds like – kirtan is about filling your heart with love, not about being a great singer or leader of singing.

JAPA, THE RECITING OF A MANTRA, AND PRAYER ■

When we say a mantra daily we can create deep, positive impressions in our mind. We can recite the mantra as part of our yoga practice, but also in our daily activities. Often in yoga schools a teacher or guru might give a mantra to us. However, we can also create our own mantras, for example, 'I am whole and loved', ' I am calm and peaceful'. Or, if you'd prefer to use a Sanskrit mantra, you could use one of the universal mantras; these include 'Om', which we've explored above, or 'So Hum', which means 'I am all that is'. To practise the 'So Hum' mantra, as you inhale, imagine you are saying the word 'So' and as you exhale, imagine you are saying the word 'Hum'. Listen to the sounds of the words on your breath and contemplate their meaning. Choose a period of time to do your mantra or japa practice, and then practise for that period of time, either aloud or silently. You can also practise for a set number of repetitions, and some people use prayer beads to help keep track of the number.

Leading on from japa is the use of prayer. We can use prayer in a number of ways, such as in an ego-centred prayer, where we tend to ask for things, but genuine prayer comes from within and will include gratitude. As mentioned earlier, to be alive on the earth is the result of an extraordinary series of events including those of our ancestors. Therefore in our prayers we should include gratitude. Leading Buddhist monk and teacher Matthieu Ricard shows that when we can cultivate a sense of gratitude, we can lead a happier and more fulfilled life (see TED 2004). If we ourselves are living with dementia or are caring for someone who is living with dementia we might feel that we do not have much to be grateful for. However, once we start to express gratitude for the little and simple things, such as clean water, sunlight, a dry place to sleep, being warm and well fed, we can open ourselves up to feeling more gratitude.

If we do not believe in an external presence we can pray to the best version of ourselves to be able to face the problems we have in our lives and do our best. Like our sankalpa (see page 234, Chapter 14, on yoga nidra), when we make an intention or prayer with genuine feeling and integrity, it is bound to be answered. Prayer is also a great way of articulating our desires and keeping focused on our needs.

LEARNING AND CONTEMPLATION

Many of the great historical teachers taught a form of bhakti yoga that is, in its essence, a practice of cultivating love and compassion for all. We can therefore use inspiring writings such as those from the Bible, Koran, Bhagavad Gita or any other inspirational book as teachings. I remember my paternal grandmother always used to read passages from the Sikh book, and as I write this I can visualise her hands as she gently turned the pages and her lips forming the words. You might also want to read other inspiring works such as the poetry of Rumi, the words of Jiddu Krishnamurti, Khalil Gibran or other great modern teachers or poets. To incorporate this into our practice we can read a short passage each day and reflect on it throughout the day, or if we are running classes for others, we can read a passage at the beginning or end of the class.

There is an impression amongst some younger people that older people do not want to learn new things and are not open to new experiences. However, in my work with an older generation I have been surprised at how receptive they are to learning and developing new skills and trying new things.

SOME OTHER IDEAS FOR CREATING MORE BHAKTI IN YOUR LIFE

As described in 'Where to practice' in Chapter 7 (see page 119), you could create a sacred space or altar in your room, or help someone you care for create one. On it you could include an image of someone inspiring or a divine figure, family members or ancestors. You could also include an inspiring book. You could put flowers or incense on the altar or make offerings of fruit. Try to make this a really beautiful space for yourself or the person you care for. You can then use it as a focus point for your prayers.

Meditate on your image of your god, whether it be the feet, hands or whole image; if you are not religious you could meditate on an image of someone who inspires you, or a symbol, word or the light of a candle flame. Visualise the image between your eyebrows. If you find it hard to visualise an image, you could use an actual image to focus on to start with, then practise closing your eyes and try to keep the image there.

Another great practice is to do a difficult or unpleasant job for someone else, or to do a task you believe someone else would not wish to do.

CONCLUSION

As you can see from these practices, I have provided a wide range of ways we can introduce more love into our lives and the lives of the people we care for. Of course it is not necessary to do all the practices outlined above; rather, I recommend trying one or two at a time and seeing how they affect you or the person or people you are helping. You could also try using your notebook to observe the patterns of your mind, emotions and practices, to reflect on where you have felt love during the day, and the things you did to cultivate it.

CHAPTER 14

YOGA, MEDITATION AND MEDITATION FOR ADVANCED STAGES OF DEMENTIA, DEATH AND DYING

This chapter provides a number of calming and soothing practices that can be done during the more advanced stages of dementia. My grandmother is currently living with late-stage dementia; she can no longer respond to people and is unable to speak or follow instructions. When speaking to people about suitable yoga for those living with dementia, they often assume that you can only do yoga when you are living with the early stages of dementia; however, you have hopefully already seen from this book that the practice of yoga encompasses many different practices, both physical and mental, that can be done throughout someone's life. This chapter provides calming practices that can be done at any stage of dementia but that are particularly suitable for those living with advanced dementia.

When someone is living with the late stages of dementia they might have lost the ability to speak, move or express their wishes, so it is important to observe and respond to their body language and expressions. Many people can still receive and return emotional signals and may be able to understand words long after they have lost the ability to speak. Therefore if you are doing yoga with someone going through the later stages of dementia, it is especially important to follow the advice given in Chapter 7 to check in with your mood and mental state before working with that person. Always speak slowly and calmly, and talk to the person normally about the practices that you are going to do.

In the later stages of dementia some people become restless because they need more physical activity. In these cases yoga is great, and if you have been working with the person for a while, you could do some of the exercises from the previous chapters. Additionally, as people become less mobile in the later stages of dementia, they have an increased risk of developing pressure sores. Yoga, by encouraging movement, can help reduce this risk. Sedentary behaviour can also lead to people developing infections and blood clots, which can be fatal. Again, active yoga movements can help, and any of the gentle movements from the previous chapters could be tried if the person is happy to do them. However, in this chapter we have focused on activities that can be done lying down or on a chair.

We also deal here with the often-ignored subject of dying. Death in modern society is rarely discussed, and for many it is seen as a taboo subject. However, each day we live, we move closer towards death. Death is a great leveller in life, as we are all at some point in the distant or not so distant future going to die. The experience of losing my father when I was 21 has taught me not to shy away from pain or talking about death. It has also helped me have open and honest conversations with friends and others who have been bereaved.

It is said that when we can be more honest about the fact we are going to die, or our relatives and friends are going to die, we can be more honest about how we live. When faced with death we can live life more fully. An example of this is an exercise that is popular amongst life coaches and self-help books. Here is a simple version.

 ## REFLECTIONS ON MORTALITY

Close your eyes and imagine you have been diagnosed with a terminal disease and you only have a year to live. What would you spend that year doing? Who would you see and how would you spend your time? Now imagine the time reducing to six months, then one month and then one week. Next, spend some time thinking about the things you do now and the things you would do if you only had a short time to live. Are there any changes you can bring into your life now to spend more time doing the things you consider important and love now? How we spend our lives is made up of the sum of the small actions and things we do on a day-to-day basis. Therefore, when we acknowledge our own death as inevitable instead of being blinded by fear of it, we can see everything else with a clearer focus, including the preciousness of every moment of life, even the moments we might think of at the time as being the bad moments.

Buddhists and others believe that things we can do to ease the suffering of those who are close to death are some of the most important actions we can take in life. Therefore this chapter brings together many things we can do to ease suffering and help people living with dementia feel calmer and well. If we can help someone who is close to death feel a bit more peaceful, then we have done a wonderful service.

Caring for someone in the later stages of dementia can be a stressful and distressing time for family members and other carers. The practices within this chapter will also help those people who are caring for the person living with dementia feel calmer and more grounded.

YOGA NIDRA

When working with people in the later stages of dementia it is recommended talking to them normally, even if they cannot respond. The natural human voice can be very soothing and help people 'get out of their own heads'. Yoga nidra is a fantastic practice for everyone, those living with dementia, caregivers and family members alike.

Yoga nidra was popularised by Swami Satyananda, and it was while living in the Satyananda ashram that I learned this practice. I found it particularly useful in times of change. Yoga nidra is sometimes thought of a type of yogic sleep, but it is actually a state somewhere between sleeping and waking, when the mind is very relaxed and open to new positive intentions known as a sankalpa. A sankalpa is a positive intention (a bit similar to a mantra, see page 30, Chapter 1) that can be used in yoga practices, meditation and yoga nidra.

To develop a sankalpa we first need to think about our lives and how we can be more true to ourselves or what we want to achieve. A sankalpa should be a long-term goal or aspiration. We should be careful of what we ask for, however, as Swami Satyananda says that our sankalpa is bound to come true (Satyananda 2001). So, for example, many people might believe that if they had more money they would be happier, or if they were slimmer they would be more fulfilled. Therefore they might think of having a sankalpa aimed at earning more or being thin. However, there may be cases when a person might get a better paid job but find that the longer hours and stress have a detrimental effect on their health. Or a person might get ill and lose a lot of weight quickly, but then not have any energy and be unable to do things. In these cases their intention would have been met, but they would not be truly any happier. In this case it would be better to have a sankalpa as something like, 'I have abundance' or 'I am healthy, vital and well'. Your sankalpa should always be phrased in positive language and be in the present tense so, instead of having phrases such as, 'I will be happy', a sankalpa should be 'I am happy'.

Don't worry if you want to try this exercise and have not yet found your sankalpa. In this case you could use the sankalpa 'I have found my path' or 'I know my true intention', and then later change it to what might come to you. If you are a carer or family member and are doing the practice with someone in the later stages of dementia you might like to take a sankalpa as well, such as 'I am loved and give love'.

Yoga nidra can be a fantastic practice to help with insomnia and other stresses.

Yoga nidra should be done from a lying down position, but can also be done from sitting back comfortably on a chair. Once lying down or sitting comfortably, all you need to do to practise yoga nidra is to listen to the instructor's voice. It is also best to cover yourself with a blanket and use a pillow. There is no need to try to analyse any of the instructions or to try to figure out what they mean; simply listen and try to remain still. There are many different variations of yoga nidra practices and many available to listen to freely on YouTube or SoundCloud. I have included a simple yoga nidra script below.

I recommend practising with a friend first, with one person reading and the other lying down. Alternatively you could record yourself reading the instructions and then listen to them. Once you have practised yoga nidra a few times, try doing it with someone living with dementia. First, make sure that the person is comfortable, relaxed and hydrated. Next, make sure their body is symmetrical either lying on the floor or sitting on a chair. Ensure their body and head is as straight as possible; you can give them a gentle adjustment if needed.

Then slowly read them the following passage, leaving lots of pauses. Keep a glass of water nearby in case your mouth gets dry.

If someone is falling asleep you can speak a little louder, but if they remain asleep, just continue to read the script as the person you are reading to might still be listening on a subconscious level.

General script for yoga nidra

This is a script for a carer or family member to read out. Alternatively you can record this script or listen to a pre-recorded yoga nidra recording.

Shortly we will be starting the practice of yoga nidra. Yoga nidra is a yogic relaxation practice that works with your subconscious mind. All you need to do is listen to my voice. Remain calm and still if you can while you listen to me talking. There is no need to over-think any of the instructions, or respond to any of the questions I ask apart from in your own mind. First, set an intention (sankalpa) for the practice. It could be something like, 'I am whole', 'I am well', or whatever intention you feel like you need today. Say to yourself, 'I am practising yoga nidra, I will try to remain awake and not move'...

Next, bring your attention to your breath, and with each out-breath see if you can feel like you are sinking deeper and deeper into the floor and relaxing more and more...

Imagine someone is pressing their finger down into the space between your eyebrows. As you feel this pressure hear your sankalpa (intention) loudly and clearly. Repeat the words to yourself in your mind, clearly listening to each one. Next, begin to listen to the sound of your inhale and exhale. See if you can feel your belly rising as you inhale and your chest releasing downwards as you exhale. Then start a slow count down from 11 to 1 as you inhale and exhale. The count down goes like this: inhale 11, exhale 11, inhale 10, exhale 10... Continue counting and breathing. Don't worry if you lose track of the counting; if you lose your place simply return to 11 and start again...

Next, take your attention to your chest and see if you can feel your breastbone lifting and falling with each breath. As you breathe in feel your chest lift, and as you breathe out feel your chest fall. Now begin counting again like this: inhale, chest lifts 11, exhale, chest falls 11. Breathe in, chest lifts 10, breathe out, chest falls 10. Continue breathing and counting with this awareness...

Wherever you are with your counting, simply leave your counting and observe your body lying gently on the floor.

Now we will begin a journey of awareness and simply move the awareness around the body. I will simply mention parts of the body and all you need to do is take your awareness to them or visualise them in your mind. There is no need to move that part of the body.

Right hand. Right-hand thumb, second finger, third finger, fourth finger, fifth finger, palm of the hand, back of the hand, wrist, forearm, elbow, upper arm, shoulder, armpit, waist, hip, thigh, knee, back of knee, shin, calf, ankle, heel, sole of the foot, top of the foot, right big toe, second toe, third toe, fourth toe, fifth toe.

Left hand. Left-hand thumb, second finger, third finger, fourth finger, fifth finger, palm of the hand, back of the hand, wrist, forearm, elbow, upper arm, shoulder, armpit, waist, hip, thigh, knee, back of knee, shin, calf, ankle, heel, sole of the foot, top of the foot, left big toe, second toe, third toe, fourth toe, fifth toe.

Now take your attention to the back of your body, right heel, left heel, right calf, left calf, right thigh, left thigh, right buttock, left buttock, lower back, middle back, upper back, the entire spine, right shoulder blade, left shoulder blade, back of the neck, back of the head.

Top of the head, forehead, right temple, left temple, right ear, left ear, right eyebrow, left eyebrow, middle of the eyebrows, right eye, left eye, eyelashes touching together, right nostril, left nostril, right cheek, left cheek, upper lip, lower lip, both lips together, chin, jaw, throat, right collarbone, left collarbone, right side of the chest, left side of the chest, upper abdomen, navel, lower abdomen, right groin, left groin, pelvic floor.

The whole right leg, whole left leg, whole right arm, whole left arm, the whole back of your body, the whole face, the whole head, the whole torso, the whole body, the whole body, the whole body...

Next, take your attention to the space behind your forehead and focus on the space in front of your closed eyelashes. Imagine this space is like a large theatre screen, that it is wide and high. Focus on this screen and become aware of any phenomena that manifests on it such as colours, patterns and light... See if you can be aware of this space but do not become involved; just observe the blank screen of the mind...

Next, I'm going to name some images... All you need to do is visualise these images... Try to engage with these images both physically and be aware of any emotional or other response. Each image will be repeated three times...don't worry if you drift off or lose focus, simply bring your attention back to my voice if you notice during the practice you have drifted off.

Beautiful garden, beautiful garden, beautiful garden...full moon, full moon, full moon...laughing with friends, laughing with friends, laughing with friends...foggy morning, foggy morning, foggy morning...a child playing on a swing, a child playing on a swing, a child playing on a swing...church bells chiming, church bells chiming, church bells chiming...cat stretching, cat stretching, cat stretching...a bright sunny day, a bright sunny day, a bright sunny day...a tall tree, a tall tree, a tall tree...a bunch of flowers, a bunch of flowers, a bunch of flowers...holding hands with someone we love, holding hands with someone we love, holding hands with someone we love...a cup of tea, a cup of tea, a cup of tea...cool clear water, cool clear water, cool clear water...birds flying across a sunrise, birds flying across a sunrise, birds flying across a sunrise...a dark starry night, a dark starry night, a dark starry night...a woman crying, a woman crying, a woman crying...a path through the woods, a path through the woods, a path through the woods...your favourite song, your favourite song, your favourite song...the sound of my voice, the sound of my voice, the sound of my voice...your body relaxing here, your body relaxing here, your body relaxing here...

Next, bring your attention back to your breath and the feeling of your body touching the ground or a chair. Take some deep breaths here. Again, imagine a finger is touching the point in between your eyebrows. At this point again remember the words of your yogic intention or sankalpa. Say the words clearly to yourself. The practice of yoga nidra is now complete.

Now take your time to get up slowly, spending a few minutes to slowly open and close your eyes. Stretch your hands and feet and slowly wake up the body.

If anyone has fallen asleep when instructing yoga nidra simply raise your voice a little louder and if necessary, gently wake them up. Check how you or the person you are working with is feeling.

HAND GESTURES, MUDRAS

When someone is living with the advanced stages of dementia it might be difficult for them to follow instructions or to do a wide range of physical movements. Therefore teaching and learning simple hand gestures can be a wonderful practice, as they can benefit even those who are bed-bound. In this section we learn two mudras or hand gestures to help improve physical, mental and spiritual wellbeing.

To help someone perform a hand mudra I first recommend giving them a simple hand massage to loosen up their joints (see page 221, Chapter 12).

Vayu mudra

The first mudra we will try is the vayu (air) mudra. This is believed to be best for people with diseases considered by the ancient Indian science of Ayurveda to be due to too much air in the body. Alzheimer's disease is considered to be such a disease as when we look at the brain of someone who has had Alzheimer's, their brain is very light and almost sponge-like due to the damaged tissue. It can also be good for anxiety and stress, so can be helpful for carers and family members alike.

This mudra can be performed sitting, standing or lying down. Fold the index finger (the first finger next to the thumb) and press the second long bone of the index finger (the middle bone) with the thumb. The tip of the index finger should touch the base of the thumb. If you are helping someone else get into the position, gently adjust their fingers into position. Allow the other fingers to remain straight.

This mudra can be practised at any time of day. I recommend practising it yourself first, and then you can help someone else practise it. As well as helping those living with dementia, it can also help to release excess gas problems and diseases such as neck pain, trembling related to Parkinson's, arthritis and balancing hormones. If helping someone else practise you can help them put both sets of hands into the right position and then stay with them for 5–10 minutes, taking slow deep breaths with them. If both hands will not stay in the position, try putting one hand into the right position and then supporting it gently with both of your hands. Do not force their hands to remain in position, and as described earlier, observe their face and breathing to ensure they remain comfortable.

Once you are comfortable with practising the vayu mudra you could also try the apana vayu mudra.

 ## Apana vayu mudra

The apana vaya mudra is said to help balance the body and is said to be great for heart health. It helps to stimulate and strengthen the blood circulation systems, the digestive system, the respiratory system and nervous system. In ancient India it was said that this mudra was given to people suffering from a heart attack as an instant remedy or rescue remedy.

This mudra has a number of benefits including helping regulate high and low blood pressure, helping to remove blockages within the veins, helping to regulate our emotions, and helping with headaches and migraines by stimulating the acupressure points in the hands and changing the flow of the subtle energy.

To do this mudra, like the first mudra, touch the index finger to the base of the thumb and then take the tip of the thumb to the middle and ring finger. The little finger should be stretched out. This mudra should be performed with both hands, if possible.

If you are helping someone living with dementia practice this mudra you could start by helping them practice it once a day for a few minutes. Over a period of weeks, gradually see if you can build up to practising the mudra 15 minutes three times a day. If you are using this mudra to help with the stress of caring you can do it anytime, for example, before bed or whilst doing something else, and you can also combine it with a restorative pose (such as legs up the wall, see page 73).

  ## SINGING MANTRAS

For someone in the late stages of dementia, another wonderful practice that you can do with them is singing mantras. Whether they can join in or not doesn't matter; the key thing is that they will be able to hear you chanting, whether consciously or subconsciously. It is also nice to hold

the hand of someone whilst you are chanting mantras, and you can, of course, also put their hand into a mudra if this is comfortable for them.

Chanting is a very personal practice, but we do not need to be a good singer or have a strong voice to be able to sing or chant. When we practice with sincerity and love, the person we are chanting with will be able to hear this in our voice.

We are now going to do a chant called 'Ra Ma Da Sa, Sa Say So Hung'. This is a beautiful chant and before we sing it we can explain to the person or people we are chanting with what the words mean. If you are uncomfortable singing by yourself you can always download a track from YouTube and sing along with it.

In this chant Raa refers to the sun and represents masculine energy. Maa represents the moon and feminine energy. Daa means the earth and represents grounding. Saa represents infinity or space and Saa Say represents the universe. So represents our self merging with infinity and Hung represents the reality of all vibrating together and everything being real.

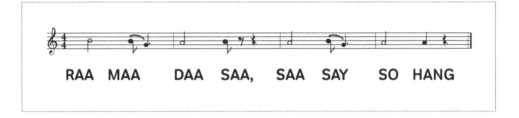

RAA MAA   DAA SAA,   SAA SAY   SO HANG

If you are not confident in singing, try searching Snatam Kaur's version on YouTube (see www.youtube.com/watch?v=kYiv P3gedCo).

GETTING READY FOR DEATH AND DYING

In Chapter 4 we looked at the fact the body is made up of a number of different sheaths or layers, know as koshas in yoga. Below we discuss these layers, and what happens when these different layers begin to dissolve.

The first layer, the annamaya kosha, represents the gross physical body. When this layer of existence dissolves the body weakens and the arms and legs become very heavy. You could do a simple head to toe guided relaxation as outlined on page 157, or a longer yoga nidra practice as outlined on page 234. The simple joint release series which begins on page 198 can be adapted to be done from lying down. Some simple mudras are outlined on page 66 and pages 239 and 240. They might appreciate being touched gently on the shoulder. At this level a person might like to connect to the water element, so, for example, they might appreciate drinking fresh, cool water, or having their hands washed with cool water.

The second layer is known as the pranamaya kosha or the energy body. Symptoms might include the lips becoming dry. At this stage a person might respond well to breathing exercises that emphasise lengthening the out-breath, or sounding a long 'ah' on the exhale, or chanting the 'sea of Oms' (see page 222, Chapter 12). You can also encourage someone to imagine they are breathing in through the skin. Yoga nidra is also very good (see page 234), as are practising dying meditations such as the four-directions meditation (see page 243). You could encourage the person to put their hand on their belly and listen to their breath.

The third layer or sheath is the manomaya kosha. During this stage it is normal for someone to have increased physical weakness, and their skin may become mottled. At this stage it is useful to take a hand on to their forehead or hold their hand. It is often good to reminisce about someone's memories and to organise visits from friends and relatives. The elements for this stage are air, so it is helpful to open a window and ensure someone has enough fresh air.

The next level is the vijnanamaya kosha; when the life leaves this sheath the skin may become slightly translucent and have a slight radiance to it. A person's breathing can be irregular, with the exhalations longer than the inhales. You might like to encourage the person you are sitting with to do some meditation. Alternatively, you could try some techniques from the previous chapter such as praying or just being. A gentle calm presence will mean a lot to the person, and a nice thing to do at this stage is just to put your hand on your client's or family member's hand and just be with them.

The last stage of the koshas, anandamaya kosha, is when we give up the final elements and enter the realms of ether, bliss, joy or peace. This is the level of surrender. At this stage a person might feel peace or gentleness surrounding them. Time might start to slow around them and the person might become more loving. They might appreciate some stories about their personal god and want to practise letting go. A nice way to practise letting go is to extend each exhale and relax each part of the body in turn (see Sequence 2 on page 151, Chapter 8). Afterwards, take one hand to your heart and join the other hand with their hand. Focus on both your heartbeats and your breath.

CYCLE OF LIFE – FOUR-DIRECTIONS MEDITATION

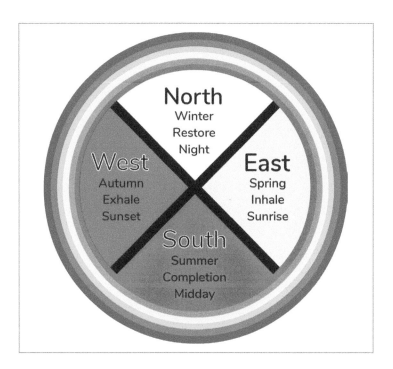

In the pagan tradition, which is grounded in respect and reverence for the natural world, calling on the four directions is the usual way to begin any ceremony. Each direction is associated with an element of the natural world, and represents some part of our human nature as well. The directions are not seen as separate and isolated, but rather as part of the interdependent system that makes up the world.

If you do not have access to the outside you might like to try this four-directions meditation and breath exercise. You can listen to this exercise on my SoundCloud link (https://soundcloud.com/taniayogini), or you can read it to those you are working with, or record yourself reading it and listen to your own voice.

Sit or lie down in a comfortable position. Let your body settle into the floor and with each exhale imagine you sinking deeper and deeper as you relax further and further. Then bring your attention to your breath, noticing your inhale, exhale and the pauses between the breaths. Allow your breath to be full and natural...

Next bring more of your attention to the in-breath. This represents the east, the rising sun, new ideas or inspiration. See if you can feel each in-breath, noticing the way it takes a bit of effort. See if you can notice the fullness of the in-breath. As you breathe in think about times of expansion in your life, of the dawn, of a new project, and new beginnings, of new life and experiences. See if you can feel that expansion on each inhale. Pause for a few breaths as you experience the inhale and the expansion. The element associated with the east is air. Air is associated with breath, which in turn gives us life. The word 'inspiration' literally means to take in air. So therefore the east is associated with new ideas, learning and inspiration. The east represents a fresh start and a new idea, which we can start with an invigorating breath. If you feel stuck, look to the east or the direction of the rising sun, or meditate on a feather, to feel unstuck.

Next, allow your attention to move to the pause after the inhale as your body is full of breath. This pause after the inhale can be linked to the southern point of the compass, to the midday and to projects completed. See if you can rest your awareness in this pause. In this stage of the breath we reap the benefits of the inhale and the oxygen in the lungs. As we focus on the inhale we can think about the satisfaction of jobs completed, of long hot summers, of the south. Take a few rounds of breath, letting the attention rest more on the pause after the inhale.

The next point of the compass is the south. The south is associated with the element of fire. Fire is hugely transformative; it burns away the old and makes way for the new. When things get cold in the northern hemisphere we move south; birds and other animals migrate to where they can live more easily and be warmer. If we feel our internal fire has cooled, focus on the element of the south, fire and the sun.

Turn your attention to the exhale. The exhale can be linked to the western point of the compass, to autumn; it is a process of letting go. See if we can find the end of the exhale and then exhale a bit further to get rid of a bit more of the stale air in the lungs. Imagine autumn and the trees letting go of their leaves. Imagine the sun setting in the west and think about things that you need to let go of. Think of projects finished and letting these go. Think of the space you can create by letting go of things that no longer serve you, and see if you can let go a bit more on each exhale.

The next point on the compass is the west. The west is associated with water. The west is associated with self-reflection and self-understanding and also letting go of what no longer serves us and following the river of life. Our emotions move and shift like water, sometimes calm and sometimes turbulent, but always changing. When water is stopped from flowing, pressure builds up and similarly, if our emotions are stopped from flowing, pressure will build. If you feel like you need to change your emotional landscape, focus on the west and change. You could imagine the sun setting over the sea or a lake.

After a few breaths take your awareness to the pause after the exhale, the place of no-breath. This pause can be equated with the north, winter or night-time. It is when in the winter on the surface of the ground not much seems to be happening, although underground lots might be happening, for example, new roots are growing, and animals might be resting or hibernating. We can equate this pause with times of our life when we had rests or pauses. We might not think much is going on in this pause but this is the place of rest or peace. The pauses are essential for the cycle of breath and the cycle of life.

We move now to the north, which is represented by earth. This earth represents stability and grounding and also stillness and silence. The north is associated with the earth that holds us, and gives us time and space to heal and grow, and to feel nurtured. It is about connecting with others, ourselves and the earth. If you are seeking balance, and a place of rest and recovery, focus on the north.

Next, see if you can take your attention to the whole cycle of life and the breath: the inhale, the pause, the exhale and the pause. See if you can follow this cycle around and imagine each part of the cycle like a point on a compass. If you find your attention wandering, see if you can use a word for each stage of the breath; for example, for the inhale you could use a word representing something you want more of, such as 'peace', 'hope' etc. For the pause after the inhale you could use a word that represents something you already have that you are grateful for, such as 'love', 'family'. For the exhale, think of something you want to let go of, such as 'fear', 'doubt'. On the pause after the exhale use a word that represents rest, such as 'peace', 'sleep', 'surrender'. On each round of breath say the words to yourself. See if you can enjoy the breath and the gentle repeating of the words.

CONCLUSION

In this chapter we have explored a sequence of restful practices for those living with all stages of dementia, but that are particularly suited to those in the later stages. These practices also help prepare ourselves, and those we are working with, for their final journey. And as explained in previous chapters, they can be performed with any personal god or nature as a focus.

CONCLUSION

When you or a loved one or a client/patient are living with dementia, it might feel like you are embarking on a scary journey. You may not know where you are going, how you will get there and what you need to take with you. You might worry about losing things on the journey or be frightened of what you may find at the end. Of course when we are unsure about a journey it is better to find out as much as we can about it, and take a map, tools and supplies to assist us on the long road ahead. We may also want to plan parts of our journey in advance.

The knowledge, sequences, tips and information you have read about in this book have been designed to provide you or your loved ones with a yogic tool kit or 'travel guide' to ease you on your way on your journey with dementia. Throughout I have demonstrated tried and tested tools and techniques, which aim to reduce the negative impacts of living with dementia, and in turn, help us improve our everyday wellbeing.

By using this book as your number one essential tool, and recording what you do in your notebook, you have begun to prepare for and chart your journey. Learning and sharing the practical yoga exercises will enable you and your loved ones to live in the moment, feel well and create more happy memories. This book will also provide you with ways of creating safe and calming environments to enable you to rest during your journey.

Taking time to pause, reflect and accept ourselves and, of course, others, is a key part of any yoga journey. Living with dementia or being with someone going through this journey has been described by carers and family members as being both the best of times, and, needless to say, the worst of times too. Being with a loved one on their journey with dementia can give us great insight into the fragility of life, and the vulnerability we all face. It can help us reflect on what is important for us, the bigger picture and our deep capacity for love and compassion. When my father died early in my life, I felt the grief of losing him hollowed me out. In the longer term this has given me more perspective and the desire not to put off focusing on my dreams, not to take simple things for granted, or to spend too much time worrying about the little things.

Writing this book has been a remarkable journey for me, too, and I am really thrilled to share the many things I have discovered along the way. As you will have experienced throughout this book there are many different combinations of poses and activities you can do and try. No two people are the same, and although if you are living with dementia you might have some common experiences, each day will be different and each person will have a different experience. We all have unique backgrounds, different bodies and varying energy levels, and choosing the appropriate sequences and activities for yourself, or those you are working with, is key to getting the most out of the book.

On the very best yogic journeys we take time to explore, so do not be afraid of trying the wide range of practices contained in this book. However, once you have found some practices you or those you are working with like, do not shy away from sticking to those that work. Often those living with dementia like a daily routine, so maybe include some key exercises as part of a daily practice, and then only add on to these once you or those you are working with feel ready to move on. Also, do not forget the importance of rest on long journeys – this book contains plenty of restful poses and relaxations.

I truly believe that simple, adapted yoga has huge potential to bring so much serenity and joy to those living with dementia, and to those who care for them. It has the potential to heal our bodies, hearts and minds through its ability to help us accept ourselves, and in understanding the interconnectivity of life. Yoga teaches that we are one, and kindness and compassion are the ultimate expressions of this understanding. I hope you can use this book to be kind to yourself and to those around you, in particular, those who are vulnerable. Caring for the vulnerable, being patient, providing activities that are stimulating but not patronising are huge challenges for an ageing society with rapidly increasing numbers of people living with dementia. Yoga provides many tools to help with this.

A conclusion is often an ending statement; however, I hope that reading this conclusion will be just part of a long and fruitful journey for you. If you have read this book from start to finish, it is likely you have learned a great deal about how yoga can help people living with dementia and those who are touched by it. I sincerely hope you feel inspired to carry on practising and also sharing what you have learned with others. For me, this book started with a vision and a dream of seeing people living with dementia engaging in stimulating and calming activities that they could do themselves or with those close to them in the comfort of their own environment. I sought to make the practices accessible and easy. If you or your loved ones have found one joyful practice or had one extra moment of peace or connection as a result of this book, I will consider my time writing and researching it well spent.

Of course I would love to hear from people about their experience with yoga, and collect further feedback and evidence about which exercises and yoga sequences were helpful for you and your loved ones. I also offer a service to help care homes implement adapted yoga sessions for their residents. For more information and to get in touch, see www.yoga4dementia.com.

■■■ GLOSSARY

Asana – means position or seat. In yoga, asana normally refers to a physical yoga position.

Ayurveda – the Indian science of health and wellbeing. A sister science to yoga.

Bhakti Yoga (Yoga of devotion) – a major branch of the yoga tradition.

Chakra – a spinning wheel of internal energy. The basic system has seven chakras (root, sacrum, solar plexus, heart, throat, eyebrow center and crown of head) each of which is associated with a particular quality, element, color, symbol, sound and significance.

Dharma – sometimes translated as 'duty' but more often as ones path or truth.

Drishti – gazing point used during asana practice.

Guru – a teacher or spiritual mentor / leader, also means one who brings light to darkness.

Karma Yoga – the yoga of action.

Karma – action or the law of cause and effect.

Kirtan – a community gathering involving chanting, live music and meditation.

Mantra – a repeated sound, syllable, word or phrase often used in chanting and meditation.

Mudra – generally refers to a specific hand or body position which again aims to change the subtle energy balance within the body.

Nadis – energy channels within the body.

Niyama – five living principles that (along with the yamas) make up the ethical and moral foundation of yoga.

Om – a sacred syllable; chanted "A-U-M" often used in yoga. Om has many meanings relating to its three syllables and is considered the most sacred mantra in Hinduism and Tibetan Buddhism.

Prana – our vital life energy or force, this is also known as chi or qi in Chinese medicine.

Pranayama – usually refers to a specific breathing exercise. Prana generally means the life force or energy and Yama or Ayama means to control or direct the energy in the body so a longer definition could be to control or direct the life force in the body.

Pranayama – exercises involving breath control which help to shift energy in the body.

Surya Namaskar – Sun Salutations; a complete system of yoga exercises performed in a specific series.

Shavasana – one of the key resting poses in yoga. It can be performed before or after any yogic pose or practice and helps to integrate the results.

Yamas – five living principles or codes of conduct that along with Niyamas make up the ethical and moral foundation of yoga.

Yogi/Yogini – a male/female practitioner of yoga.

■■■ REFERENCES

Alzheimer's Association (2015) *Dementia Facts and Figures: A Special Report.* Accessed on 1/6/2017 at www.alz.org/facts/downloads/facts_figures_2015.pdf

Alzheimer's Association (2016) *2016 Alzheimer's Disease Facts and Figures.* Accessed on 1/6/2017 at www.alz.org/documents_custom/2016-facts-and-figures.pdf

Alzheimer's Association (n.d.) *Mild Cognitive Impairment.* Accessed on 3/3/2017 at www.alz.org/dementia/mild-cognitive-impairment-mci.asp

Alzheimer's Research UK (2015) 'One in three people born in 2015 will develop dementia, new analysis shows.' Accessed on 1/6/2017 at www.alzheimersresearchuk.org/one-in-three-2015-develop-dementia/

American Psychological Association (n.d.) *Aging and Depression.* Accessed on 3/3/2017 at www.apa.org/helpcenter/aging-depression.aspx

Ammachi (n.d.) www.beliefnet.com/wellness/2008/11the-wisdom-of-amma.aspx/p=2

Balasubramaniam, M., Telles, S. and Doraiswamy, P. (2012) 'Yoga on our minds: A systematic review of yoga for neuropsychiatric disorders.' *Frontiers in Psychiatry 3*, 117.

Bilderbeck, A., Farias, M., Brazil, I., Jakobowitz, S. and Wikholm, C. (2013) 'Participation in a 10-week course of yoga improves behavioural control and decreases psychological distress in a prison population.' *Journal of Psychiatric Research 47*, 10, 1438–1445.

Caitlin, A. (2015) 'The role of massage therapy in dementia care.' *Massage Today 15*, 4. Accessed on 1/6/2017 at www.massagetoday.com/mpacms/mt/article.php?id=15057

Centers for Disease Control and Prevention Newsroom (2014) 'Up to 40 percent of annual deaths from each of five leading US causes are preventable.' Accessed on 22/08/2017 at https://www.cdc.gov/media/releases/2014/p0501-preventable-deaths.html

Chiesa, A. and Serretti, A. (2009) 'Mindfulness-based stress reduction for stress management in healthy people: A review and meta-analysis.' *Journal of Alternative and Complementary Medicine 15*, 5, 593–600.

Dusek, J., Otu, H., Wohlhueter, A., Bhasin, M., Zerbini, L., Joseph, M., *et al.* (2008) 'Genomic counter-stress changes induced by the relaxation response.' *PLoS ONE 3*, 7.

Eyre, H. A., Acevedo, B., Yang, H., Siddarth, P., van Dyk, K., Ercoli, L., *et al.* (2016) 'Changes in neural connectivity and memory following a yoga intervention for older adults: A pilot study.' *Journal of Alzheimer's Disease 52*, 673–684.

Farhi, D. (1996) *The Breathing Book: Good Health and Vitality Through Essential Breath.* New York: Holt Paperbacks.

Fredrickson, B., Cohn, M., Coffey, K., Pek, J. and Finkel, S.M. (2008) 'Open hearts build lives: Positive emotions, induced through loving-kindness meditation, build consequential personal resources.' *Journal of Personality and Social Psychology 95*, 5, 1045–1062.

Golubic, M. (2013) *Lifestyle Choices: Root Causes of Chronic Diseases.* Accessed on 22/2/2017 at https://my.clevelandclinic.org/health/transcripts/1444_lifestyle-choices-root-causes-of-chronic-diseases

Goel. A. (n.d.) 'Cool down this Summer with Sheetali Pranayama.' *Health and Yoga.* Accessed on 1/6/2017 at www.healthandyoga.com/html/news/sheetali.aspx

Gu, S., Zhang, Y. and Wu, Y. (2016) Effects of sound exposure on the growth and intracellular macromolecular synthesis of *E. coli* k-12. *PeerJ 4*, e1920.

Hanford, N. and Figueiro, M. (2013) 'Light therapy and Alzheimer's disease and related dementia: Past, present, and future.' *Journal of Alzheimer's Disease 33*, 4, 913–922.

Hartfiel, N., Burton, C., Rycroft-Malone, J., Clarke, G., Havenhand, J., Khalsa, S. and Edwards, R. (2012) 'Yoga for reducing perceived stress and back pain at work.' *Occupational Medicine 62*, 8, 606–612.

Headly, G. (2009) *Fascia and Stretching: The Fuzz Speech.* [video]. Accessed on 1/6/2017 at www.youtube.com/watch?v=_FtSP-tkSug

Hobson, H. (2013) *10 Foods that Prevent Dementia and Alzheimer's.* MindBodyGreen. Accessed on 1/1/2017 at www.mindbodygreen.com/0-7613/10-foods-that-prevent-dementia-alzheimers.html

Jenkinson, S. (2015) *Die Wise: A Manifesto for Sanity and Soul.* Berkeley, CA: North Atlantic Books.

Kassaar, O., Pereira Morais, M., Xu, S., Adam, E., Chamberlain, R., Jenkins, B. *et al.* (2017) 'Macrophage migration inhibitory factor is subjected to glucose modification and oxidation in Alzheimer's Disease.' *Scientific Reports 7*, 42874.

McCall, T. (2007) *Yoga as Medicine: The Yogic Prescription for Health and Healing.* New York: Bantam Dell.

Moss, M., Hewitt, S., Moss, L. and Wesnes, K. (2008) 'Modulation of cognitive performance and mood by aromas of peppermint and ylang-ylang.' *International Journal of Neuroscience 188*, 1.

NICE (National Institute for Care and Excellence) (2015) *Physical Activity for NHS Staff, Patients and Carers.* Accessed on 1/1/2017 at www.nice.org.uk/guidance/qs84/chapter/introduction

Ornish, D., Lin, J., Chan, J., Epel, E., Kemp, C., Weidner, G., *et al.* (2013) 'Effect of comprehensive lifestyle changes on telomerase activity and telomere length in men with biopsy-proven low-risk prostate cancer: 5-year follow-up of a descriptive pilot study.' *Lancet Oncology 14*, 11, 1112–1120.

Parnetti, L. and Calabresi, P. (2006) 'Spatial cognition in Parkinson's disease and neurodegenerative dementias.' *Cognitive Processing 7*, Suppl. 1, 77.

Pomykala, K., Silverman, D., Geist, C., Voege, P., Siddarth, P., Nazarian, N., *et al.* (2012) 'A pilot study of the effects of meditation on regional brain metabolism in distressed dementia caregivers.' *Aging Health 8*, 5, 509–516.

Ross, A. and Thomas, S. (2010) 'The health benefits of yoga and exercise: A review of comparison studies.' *The Journal of Alternative and Complementary Medicine 16*, 1, 3–12.

Särkämö, T., Tervaniemi, M., Laitinen, S., Numminen, A., Kurki, M., Johnson, J. and Rantanen, P. (2014) 'Cognitive, emotional, and social benefits of regular musical activities in early dementia: Randomized controlled study.' *Gerontologist 54*, 4, 634–650.

Satyananda, S. (2001) *Yoga Nidra.* Munger, Bihar, India: Yoga Publications Trust.

Saunders, G. and Echt, K. (2007) 'An overview of dual sensory impairment in older adults: Perspectives for rehabilitation.' *Trends in Amplification 11*, 4, 243–258.

Tang, Y., Hölzel, B. and Posner, M. (2015) 'The neuroscience of mindfulness meditation.' *Nature Reviews. Neuroscience 16*, 4, 213–225.

TED (2004) *Matthieu Ricard: The Habits of Happiness* [video]. Accessed on 1/1/2017 at www.ted.com/talks/matthieu_ricard_on_the_habits_of_happiness?language=en

Telles, S. (2016) *The Basis and Application of Yoga for Healthy Aging.* Accessed on 22/2/2017 at www.iayt.org/resource/resmgr/docs_syr2016/07_Telles-keynote.pdf

Tran, M.D., Holly, R.G., Lashbrook, J. and Amsterdam, E.A. (2001) 'Effects of Hatha yoga practice on the health-related aspects of physical fitness.' *Preventive Cardiology 4*, 165–170.

Whitson, H., Johnson, K., Sloane, R., Cigolle, C., Pieper, C., Landerman, L. and Hastings, S. (2016) 'Identifying patterns of multimorbidity in older Americans: Application of latent class analysis.' *Journal of the American Geriatrics Society 64*, 8, 1668–1673.

■■■ FURTHER READING AND RESOURCES

This book contains a wealth of resources and has adapted the best techniques from a number of yoga schools to provide all you need to embark on your yoga journey. Yogic knowledge is really very vast and has many paths of enquiry, and I hope you will find much joy and knowledge through your practice and explorations. If you would like to delve deeper and want some recommendations for further reading, here are a few of my favourite traditional and modern yoga reference books.

Satyananda Saraswati, S. (2008) *Asana Pranayama Mudra Bandha*. Munger, Bihar, India: Yoga Publications Trust (Original work published in 1969). This is a fantastic book full of lots of useful information about yoga, mudras, breathing techniques and internal awareness techniques. It is a great resource if you have read this book and want to delve more into general yoga.

Satyananda Saraswati, S. (2001) *Yoga Nidra*. Munger, Bihar, India: Yoga Publications Trust. If you or those you are working with enjoyed the yoga nidra practices in my book and want to find out more, I strongly recommend reading this excellent book.

Farhi, D. (1996) *The Breathing Book: Good Health and Vitality Through Essential Breath.* New York: Holt Paperbacks. If you enjoyed the breathing exercises within this book, I thoroughly recommend Donna Farhi's book. The simple and effective breathing practices contained within this book really helped me discover the joy of full and deep breathing.

Iyengar, B.K.S. (1966; revised edn 1977) *Light on Yoga*. New York: Schocken. This is a large and comprehensive book for those who enjoyed the yoga asanas and feel able to and want to try more physical positions. It contains hundreds of poses and detailed instructions on how to do them.

McCall, T. (2007) *Yoga as Medicine: The Yogic Prescription for Health and Healing*. New York: Bantam Dell. This is a great book for healthcare workers and yoga teachers who might want to learn more about the healing power of yoga.

Colouring Books Now (2016) *Simple Mandala Coloring Book for Adults: Stress Relief Coloring Book for Grown Ups Including Over 40 Easy Mandalas Designed for Beginners*. CreateSpace Independent Publishing Platform. If you or those you work with enjoy the mandala practices in Chapter 3, this is a great little book for doing some more relaxing colouring.

Girish (2016) *Music and Mantras: The Yoga of Mindful Singing for Health, Happiness, Peace & Prosperity*. New York: Atria Books. If you found the singing practices enjoyable and would like to explore this part of yoga more, I recommend this book by one of my favourite kirtan artists. If you are unsure about the book you could always have a look and listen to some of his songs on YouTube.

■■■ INDEX